HOSPITAL-PHYSICIAN RELATIONSHIPS

Case Studies and Commentaries on Medical Staff Problems

HOSPITAL-PHYSICIAN RELATIONSHIPS

Case Studies and Commentaries on Medical Staff Problems

Nathan Hershey, LL.B.
Editor and Contributing Author

AN ASPEN PUBLICATION®
Aspen Systems Corporation
Rockville, Maryland
London
1982

Library of Congress Cataloging in Publication Data
Main entry under title:

Hospital-physician relationships.

1. Hospitals—Medical staff—Case studies.
2. Hospitals—Administration—Case studies.
3. Medical laws and legislation—United States—Case studies. I. Hershey, Nathan.
[DNLM: 1. Medical staff, Hospital.
2. Physicians. 3. Public relations.
4. Governing board. 5. Interprofessional relations. WX 160 H828]
RA972.H68 1982 362.1'1'0683 82-11359
ISBN: 0-89443-386-5

Publisher: John Marozsan
Editorial Director: Mike Brown
Managing Editor: Margot Raphael
Editorial Services: M. Eileen Higgins
Printing and Manufacturing: Debbie Collins

Library of Congress Catalog Card Number: 82-11359
ISBN: 0-89443-386-5

Printed in the United States of America

1 2 3 4 5

This book is dedicated
to all the members of the hospital community—
physicians, executives, nurses, and other personnel—
and to the attorneys who serve that community.

Table of Contents

Acknowledgments

The editor gratefully acknowledges the contributions of the authors: Walter Cheifetz, of Lewis and Roca, Phoenix; Frank R. Ciesla, of Giordano, Halleran, & Crahay, Middletown, N.J.; Wayne J. Fowler, of Saunders, Snyder, Ross, & Dickson, P.C., Denver; Gladys George, legal counsel, Lenox Hill Hospital, New York; George Huber, assistant director and legal counsel, Western Psychiatric Institute and Clinic, Pittsburgh; and Dennis J. Purtell, of Purtell, Purcell, Wilmot, & Burroughs, Milwaukee. Without their willingness to devote considerable time and effort, this volume could not have been created.

The editor further acknowledges with appreciation the editorial assistance of his wife, Carol Hershey, and the secretarial services of Dawna Baird and Ann Thomas, in the preparation of the manuscript.

Introduction

The relationships of the individual practicing physician and of the organized medical staff to the hospital, as represented by its governing board and chief executive officer, have evolved remarkably in the last 20 or so years. The pressures leading to change have been many and varied. The relationships will continue to evolve as governmental intervention in the health industry increases and as techniques for assessing the need for, and quality of, medical services become more valid and reliable.

The response to these pressures has resulted in part in the imposition of controls and limitations upon decision making by individual doctors and has brought the hospital as an institution to involve itself more in the direction and assessment of physician performance. These intrusions into various aspects of medical practice, asserted to be necessary to fulfill obligations for public accountability imposed on hospitals, are distressing to many physicians, not so much for what they have done to medical practitioners so far but for what they portend for the future.

Many physicians believe—and there is some evidence to support their belief—that the private entrepreneurial practice of medicine is on an irreversible downward course and that they no longer will be their own masters.

There are some who relish the thought that physicians and their staff organizations are losing power in hospitals. If this be true, who is exercising the power that the physicians have lost, and how is it being done? Is the public being better served now by the health industry generally, and the medical profession particularly, as physician domination erodes and power passes into the hands of others?

Organized medicine, state medical licensing boards, and medical educators are largely on the defensive today, assailed by critics in and out of government who charge all manner of conduct contrary to the public interest. But it is the practicing physicians who comprise the organized hospital medical staffs, rather than the county, state, and national physician organizations, the state medical boards, the medical educators, and the Joint Commission on Accreditation of Hospitals, who, within the profession, still largely determine the nature of medicine as it is practiced day to day in private offices and institutions, within the larger context of governmental and other types of societal regulation.

The hospital medical staff has responsibilities that have been thrust upon it that call for it to monitor, assess, and control physician performance. When the medical staff meets these responsibilities, the possibility for conflict with individual physicians is great. When the staff does not meet them and the hospital seeks to have them met nonetheless, additional bases for conflict are created. There also are circumstances when either medical staffs or hospitals abuse their powers by arbitrary or capricious decisions under the guise of fulfilling their responsibilities. These decisions breed conflict as well.

Federal and state law developments have affected hospital-medical staff relations generally, and the rights of institutions and physicians particularly, when physicians' obtaining and maintaining access to facilities crucial to their practice are at stake. The law governing hospital-medical staff relations has developed rapidly in the last 25 years. The broad range of issues and the volume of controversies concerning these relations account for the legislation and court decisions on the subject that appear with increasing frequency.

While the nature of the hospital relationships with individual physicians and staff organizations in the future cannot be predicted with certainty, views of physicians—both individually and collectively as medical staffs—of their prerogatives and responsibilities cannot always be in harmony with the attitudes of the hospital as an entity with its own prerogatives and responsibilities.

The objective of this volume is to acquaint hospital executives, hospital board members, physicians, and hospital attorneys with some of the dimensions of the problems in these relationships. Court decisions do not convey the intricacies, the role of personalities, the impact of institutional commitments to the general public and to specific constituencies, and other factors that both engender controversies and bring about specific resolutions. Even the transcripts of proceedings conducted in the hospital and in court, together with all the records and memoranda, often do not provide the entire picture. Without the "inside story," as it might be called, the full range of considerations that influence the handling of a medical staff controversy cannot be known or understood.

The method of approach here is to take some typical factual situations arising in the context of hospital-medical staff relationships and to explore them in detail. The objective is to better understand the issues—the obvious and the not so obvious—and the nature of the resolution of the conflicts in these situations.

All of these case studies are fiction. Any resemblance to actual persons and events is purely coincidental. The case studies include the inside story as well as the surface events that would have been before the court if, or when, litigation took place in such situations. Each case is followed by a commentary prepared by the author and the editor.

The authors and the editor hope that, from these case studies and commentaries, readers will gain insights that will make it possible for intelligence and rationality to have fuller play so that future controversies can be handled more skillfully or can be avoided. This is not to suggest that in all circumstances when conflict is present, going to the mat (or to the court) can or should be avoided. Rather, it is to assist people in the hospital field to understand better when confrontation is necessary and when it may be avoided.

It is not surprising that case studies and commentaries written by lawyers frequently refer to the failure to involve the hospital attorney in the situation more promptly. A parallel in medicine is the often expressed statement by physicians that if the patient had sought medical care sooner the condition would have been controlled or cured more easily and quickly.

Medical staff conflicts are traumatic for all concerned. If it is possible to learn from the experiences of others, as the authors and editor devoutly believe, then the preparation of these case studies and commentaries will have been well worth the effort expended in writing them.

Nathan Hershey
August 1982

Case 1

A Conflict between Physicians Becomes a Medical Staff Controversy

PERSONAE

Dr. Frank Archer and Dr. Ralph Baker, partners and protagonists
Dr. Miles Carter, orthopedist and protagonist
Dr. Julian Meyer, physician who died
Dr. Martin Frank, president of the staff, Hospital Y
Dr. Robert Fuller, orthopedist on Executive Committee
Benjamin Harris, president of the board of Hospital Y
Chris Lewis, attorney for Dr. Carter
Harry Long, attorney for Hospital Y
Dr. William Richards, chairman of Pediatrics Department
Dr. William Robin, chairman of Orthopedics Department
Carlton Trask, member of board and of hearing committee
Dr. Stanley Webb, internist on Executive Committee
John Wood, Hospital Y administrator

Drs. Frank Archer and Ralph Baker were partners in the practice of orthopedics. They were successful enough to conclude that it would be advantageous to recruit a young physician to join their practice. Dr. Archer was in his early 50s and Dr. Baker his late 40s. They reasoned that, with the practice growing slowly but steadily, adding a physician would enable them to avoid increasing the time they devoted to patients, yet continue to expand office volume.

An opportunity to add a third physician presented itself in 1969 and an offer was made to, and accepted by, a young orthopedic surgery resident who was completing his training at the hospital where they conducted most of their practice. Dr. Miles Carter, the young orthopedist, was hired for a salary of $20,000 and was given to understand orally that, if the practice continued to grow and his work was satisfactory, he would be given an opportunity to buy in and become a partner. He signed a contract of employment with the partnership and began practice with Drs. Archer and Baker immediately upon completion of his residency.

The partners held medical staff appointments at hospitals X, Y, and Z. Hospital X was a community hospital of modest reputation. Drs. Archer and Baker performed about 40 percent of their surgery there. Hospital Y was a major teaching hospital affiliated with the local medical school but had strong community ties as well. Drs. Archer and Baker, along with most of the members of the medical staff at hospital Y, had some type of clinical faculty status at the medical school, and several staff members were rather heavily engaged in the school's graduate training program. The partners, long-time members of the medical staff at hospital Y, conducted the rest of their practice there. Hospital Z was the primary affiliated teaching hospital of the medical school. The two orthopedists had courtesy category medical staff appointments at hospital Z but never admitted patients there.

When the partnership employed Dr. Carter, he quickly acquired a medical staff appointment at each of the three hospitals. Unlike the partners, Dr. Carter took advantage of the opportunity to use the facilities of hospital Z. His practice was divided among all three, with about 20 percent at hospital X, 50 percent at hospital Y, and 30 percent at hospital Z.

Within a year, Dr. Carter developed a substantial following, represented largely by referrals from physicians who had known him at hospital Y during his training, some of whom also were on the staff of hospital Z and conducted some of their practices there. The partnership's practice was growing more rapidly than Drs. Archer and Baker had even hoped because of Dr. Carter's drawing power.

For his second year of employment Dr. Carter was given a substantial raise, and intimations that he soon would be given the opportunity to join the partnership became more frequent. At the end of his second year, Dr. Carter received another substantial salary increase. The partnership's revenue continued to grow rapidly. Eight months into his third year, a prominent orthopedist in his early 50s who practiced primarily at hospital Y died suddenly of a heart attack. This physician, Dr. Julian Meyer, was a solo practitioner with a high-volume practice. The day following his death, his widow telephoned Dr. Carter and asked whether he would see patients who were scheduled by Dr. Meyer's office so the practice would be maintained in some fashion until she could dispose of it.

The young orthopedist had held Dr. Meyer in great esteem and had benefitted from his counsel during his residency so he readily agreed to see these patients several evenings a week on an indefinite basis until the widow could sell the practice. Although Mrs. Meyer offered to compensate Dr. Carter, he refused and took on this additional burden without remuneration. After two weeks he proposed to Drs. Archer and Baker that he become a partner and that the partnership purchase Dr. Meyer's practice. He told the partners that, while successful as a practitioner, Dr. Meyer had not made particularly good financial arrangements for his family's future. Dr. Carter believed that acquisition of this practice would enhance the partnership and, at the same time, allow the widow to sell it quickly at a reasonable price.

Drs. Archer and Baker told Dr. Carter they would consider the proposal. He continued to see Dr. Meyer's patients and maintain the practice. For those who required additional hospital services, including surgery, he arranged for the billing to be made on behalf of the Archer and Baker partnership, with the agreement of the widow. With respect to the office practice itself, he continued to assign the payments for the benefit of Meyer's practice. During the next several weeks, although he talked individually with both Drs. Archer and Baker, he could obtain no commitment from either one to purchase the Meyer practice or to make any definite statement as to what they intended to do. Preserving the practice under the current arrangement was becoming a great burden to Dr. Carter.

* * * * *

Then, one day, Dr. Archer abruptly told Dr. Carter that he no longer was to cover Dr. Meyer's office and should devote his full time and energy to the partnership. The young orthopedist responded that he was not neglecting the partnership's practice and that he didn't think that restricting him was fair to Dr. Meyer's widow. Furthermore, he said he was free to spend his time when he was not busy with the partnership's patients in any way he wanted. Dr. Archer was quite upset and reiterated his command that Dr. Carter cease his involvement with the Meyer practice. Dr. Carter asked whether the partnership was prepared to purchase the practice and Dr. Archer said "it wasn't necessary."

That evening Dr. Carter spoke with Mrs. Meyer about purchasing the practice and withdrawing from his arrangement with Drs. Archer and Baker. The widow, who had not yet been able to dispose of the practice, was thrilled and she and Dr. Carter entered into negotiations.

Dr. Carter then telephoned Dr. Archer and informed him he planned to leave the partnership at the end of his contract year, which had only about 10 weeks to run, and that he was going to purchase the Meyer practice. Dr. Archer then told Carter that he no longer was employed by them because he was engaging in medical practice that was not to the benefit of the partnership. At this point Dr. Carter concluded that the two had been relying on continuing dissipation of Dr. Meyer's practice and fully expected that, without purchasing it, they would be able to acquire it piece by piece as patients sought out the partnership as a substitute. Dr. Carter's efforts evidently were delaying the complete collapse of Dr. Meyer's practice.

Dr. Carter promptly completed his deal with the widow and began practicing full time at Dr. Meyer's old office. Meanwhile, he was being considered for annual reappointment at hospitals X and Y. He learned from friends on the staff of the former that the partners, who had considerable weight in the Department of Surgery—particularly in the orthopedic surgery section—had obtained the agreement of the department leadership to recommend that he not be reappointed. He also learned that Drs. Archer and Baker were attempting to do the same thing at hospital Y. Drs. Archer and Baker, as members of the courtesy staff at hospital Z, the primary teaching hospital of the medical school, played no role in the department so Dr. Carter's practice opportunities were not in jeopardy there.

Furthermore, while medical staff appointments at hospitals X and Y were on a fiscal year basis and the year was nearing its end, those at hospital Z were on a calendar year basis, and December was many months away, so reappointment there was not an issue. However, he could not maintain his practice entirely at hospital Z because of his low position on the seniority ladder, which largely determined elective admissions, although he was an active participant in its orthopedics training program and was well regarded by the staff.

Dr. Carter realized he was in serious danger. Loss of appointments at hospitals X and Y would restrict him to hospital Z, which could not fully meet his needs. He considered making application to the staffs of several other community hospitals but, because of travel distances and the lack of contacts that would lead to referrals, none of them were attractive settings for his practice.

At this point, he decided to seek legal advice as to his status at hospitals X and Y. He met with Chris Lewis, an attorney friend who was somewhat familiar with hospital medical staff matters. The attorney questioned him closely to learn where Dr. Carter wanted to base his practice. The orthopedist explained that hospital X, the community hospital without a teaching program, was not very attractive to him. He added that Drs. Archer and Baker had the most power to affect his medical staff appointment at hospital X.

The attorney suggested he draft a letter for Dr. Carter to send to the administrator of hospital X in which he would announce his intention to terminate his practice there at the end of the current medical staff year and express his appreciation for the past opportunities provided him. Lewis explained that withdrawing from that staff would eliminate the possibility of the hospital's taking an adverse action against him, and that he would not at some time in the future have to explain why his appointment had not been renewed there. This letter was drafted, signed, and mailed the next day.

Lewis and Dr. Carter next turned to the problem at hospital Y. It was evident that the young orthopedist needed to retain his appointment there. They agreed that he had to establish some support among the members of the department and other physicians on the staff who were making an increasing number of referrals to him. This would counteract the pressure that the partners, as long-time staff members, could bring to bear. During the almost three years of Dr. Carter's association he had become recognized as a very competent orthopedic surgeon, and some cases that in the past would have been referred to Drs. Archer and Baker as individuals had been given specifically to him because of the confidence reposed in him.

The next day he discussed the situation with several friends on the staff of hospital Y. He told them how he had covered Dr. Meyer's practice without remuneration and that some compensation for services he provided to those patients, with the widow's consent, had been directed to the Archer and Baker partnership. He also mentioned that he had proposed that the partnership acquire Dr. Meyer's practice and that this had been rejected. Most of the physicians with whom he talked were very sympathetic and offered to do what they could so he could remain a member of the staff.

Meanwhile, Drs. Archer and Baker informed their colleagues in the Department of Orthopedics that, since Dr. Carter had left their practice, there was no reason he should be retained on the hospital Y staff. Furthermore, they asserted that there already were "enough orthopedic surgeons on the staff of hospital Y" and that he was not necessary. Dr. Archer also suggested that Dr. Carter had not always practiced satisfactorily and that his ethical behavior left something to be desired.

* * * * *

Several days after the partnership terminated Dr. Carter, Dr. Archer visited the administrator of hospital Y, John Wood, and informed him that Dr. Carter had left the pair and had acquired Dr. Meyer's practice. Dr. Archer also stated that in their agreement, Dr. Carter had agreed to a restriction upon his practice if he were to leave the partnership. Dr. Archer told Wood that the hospital should not reappoint Dr. Carter because the younger physician's continued practice in the area and at hospital Y constituted a breach of the agreement with the partnership.

The administrator did not commit himself in any way, saying only that he "would look into the matter very carefully." Dr. Archer also made some thinly veiled hints that he and Dr. Baker might consider shifting a large part of their practice to hospital X where, as he put it, "we are very well liked and greatly appreciated."

Immediately after Dr. Archer left, Wood called hospital Y's attorney, Harry Long. Long was a member of a large firm that had had a prolonged association with the hospital; for 50 years, at least one firm partner had served on the hospital board. Wood described in considerable detail his conversation with Dr. Archer. After he had finished, Long asked whether Dr. Archer had shown the administrator a copy of the contract between Dr. Carter and the partnership, particularly the restriction on competition provision. Wood said that he had seen no papers and was merely reporting the substance of the conversation.

Wood asked whether the hospital had any responsibility to make a decision on medical staff appointment because of a contractual restriction of the nature that Dr. Archer asserted existed. Long replied that the hospital had to make its own decision on medical staff appointments and that if Drs. Archer and Baker were entitled to enforce a covenant in the contract that Dr. Carter would not compete, they could seek their remedies in court. The attorney added that, "there is no responsibility on the part of the hospital to make any decisions regarding Dr. Carter's medical staff status for the purpose of assisting Drs. Archer and Baker in their dispute with Carter."

"Under developing medical staff law," Long said, "a denial of appointment to Dr. Carter solely because of a contractual obligation that might or might not exist between him and Drs. Archer and Baker might very well be deemed an unreasonable decision that would allow Dr. Carter to prevail in litigation against the hospital."

Long instructed Wood to ask Dr. Archer for a copy of the contract if the subject was raised again.

The administrator was somewhat upset by the situation the hospital was in. Drs. Archer and Baker were long-standing and respected members of the medical staff and he believed their volume of admissions to the hospital was substantial. Wood decided to investigate further to determine what, if any, leverage they might be able to use against the hospital as to their admission volume. To his surprise, Wood found that their admissions had declined considerably in the last three years, although those by the partnership, if Dr. Carter's were included, had increased. Evidently, Dr. Carter was responsible for the increase in the partnership's volume of service at the hospital.

Wood then called Long, related the information he had gathered, and discussed the admissions situation. When pressed by the attorney, Wood said:

"If Dr. Carter were to be reappointed and Drs. Archer and Baker were then to decide to take all their practice elsewhere, the net effect upon admissions in orthopedics probably would be relatively small. Between the following that Dr. Carter has built up in the staff and the practice that he has acquired because of Dr. Meyer's death, we might anticipate that within a year, even if Drs. Archer and Baker reduced their practice here to a minimum, the impact would be negligible."

Long said this information was very useful.

Wood then called the chairman of the Department of Orthopedics, Dr. William Robin, and asked him to stop by his office to discuss a medical staff problem that he saw coming to a head soon. He did not indicate that it concerned the situation arising from Dr. Carter's leaving the Archer and Baker partnership.

When Dr. Robin arrived, Wood told him of the visit from Dr. Archer and asked the chairman's opinion as to the recommendation the department would make to the medical staff's Executive Committee on Dr. Carter's reappointment. Dr. Robin clearly was discomfited by the question. He paused for a moment, seeming to search for an answer, then said:

"This business of Dr. Carter's reappointment will be a real problem. Personally, from what I have seen, he has been doing a pretty good job. He attends the departmental meetings faithfully and he has relatively few surgical complications. I haven't seen anything to indicate problems with the utilization committee, and if it were my decision alone, I would recommend that he be reappointed.

"However, some of the boys, particularly Drs. Archer and Baker who are on the outs with Dr. Carter, don't believe we should have him around any more. And, as you know, according to the bylaws of the medical staff, if someone has been on the associate staff for three years, which Dr. Carter has been since his appointment, and is not recommended for promotion to the active staff, he cannot be reappointed, and that means he is out. We are meeting the night after next to make the reappointment recommendations and I frankly can't tell how it is going to turn out."

Wood, pursuing the matter, asked, "Would you go along with a vote not to promote Dr. Carter to the active staff and, if not, would you write a dissenting report if the majority voted to recommend that he not be promoted?"

Dr. Robin thought for a minute, then said, "I can't say right now what I am going to do. I have known Drs. Archer and Baker for a long time and when Dr. Archer was chairman of the department several years back he was very good to me. Besides, Dr. Carter has privileges at two other hospitals and I don't believe he would be hurt very much if he didn't practice here anymore."

The two discussed the matter further and then, as he was leaving, the department chairman said, "I hope you won't tell anybody about our conversation. I was being candid with you and I don't want to get in the middle of any disputes. I'm inclined to go along with the majority. That is the way we have done things in orthopedics since I have been around here."

Wood didn't want the conversation to end with an implication that he could not talk to anyone about what he had learned. He said:

"You realize that if your department votes to recommend that he not be promoted, and the Executive Committee does the same, and Dr. Carter wants a hearing, we are going to have to let this situation get on the table. I have already talked with Harry Long, our attorney, and I must be sure that the hospital is protected. I don't think I can talk to Long about how we deal with this without letting him know your feelings on the matter.

"I don't want to tell you what to do at the meeting, but I know you realize that we are going to have some trouble whether Dr. Carter stays on the staff or leaves. If he stays, Drs. Archer and Baker may make some waves. If he is going to be forced out, he may fight, and you have to remember that he has some friends—not only some of Dr. Meyer's old friends but also some other doctors who think he is a damn good surgeon, and better than Drs. Archer and Baker. Besides, some of the people who like Dr. Carter know some of the members of the board, and I wouldn't be surprised if they exert a little pressure there."

Dr. Robin said he understood the administrator's position and hoped there was a way to prevent Dr. Carter's reappointment from disrupting the staff and the hospital. The two shook hands and the orthopedics chairman left. Wood called Long immediately to pass on what he had learned. He described the essence of Dr. Robin's views and the difficult position the chairman felt he was in.

Long then asked, "Do you think, based on what I've told you and what else you know, that the hospital's interest will be well served if Dr. Carter is bumped from the staff, or at least put in the position where he has to fight to stay on, given the fact that there is a substantial amount of support for him on the medical staff?"

"I would hate to see Dr. Carter pushed off the staff even if he doesn't sue or even make a fuss," Wood answered.

"I really shouldn't be telling you what I am going to say now, but I think that you have to make a decision about the role you are going to play," Long said. "If I were in your shoes, I would set the stage now for the steps that would follow a negative recommendation about Dr. Carter from the department so that the end result would be that the board reappoints him. Then the ball would be in Dr. Archer's and Dr. Baker's court. If, as you told me earlier, losing them isn't going to make much of an impact on your occupancy and Dr. Carter probably is a superior practitioner to the partners, why the hell should the hospital not be encouraging Dr. Carter to stay, rather than going along with these two, who are just trying to maintain their economic situation and keep him from competing with them?"

Wood responded, "Well, you know from the bylaws, if there is a negative recommendation from the department to the Executive Committee of the staff, the Executive Committee then considers that and, in turn, makes its own recommendation to the governing board about reappointment or, as in this case, promotion to the active staff."

"If the Executive Committee submits a negative recommendation," the administrator continued, "Dr. Carter has the right to request a hearing by a committee composed of three members of the governing board and three members of the staff's Executive Committee, at which he can explain why he believes the recommendation is uncalled for or incorrect. I think he probably would request the hearing at that stage and I think it could be very embarrassing to Drs. Archer and Baker unless they have something on him that we don't know about. I guess I could talk to some members of the Executive Committee to see whether they are willing to make a recommendation contrary to that of the department in the event that the two have the votes at the meeting."

"The last thing we want to do is let this situation go to court and have all this crap about the partnership trying to keep Dr. Carter out get into the newspapers," the attorney said. "If this is supposed to be a high-quality hospital with a teaching program, we are going to look pretty silly dropping a guy from the staff who spent several years in training here.

"I don't want to tell you exactly what to do, but I hope you can arrange for the Executive Committee to recommend that he be promoted to active. If it won't go along with that, arrange that its members and those of the governing board who would be selected to participate in the hearing are people who would be sympathetic to Dr. Carter. That way I think we can head off any serious embarrassment. I don't want to tell you how to run the hospital but you know how to pass the word around. I know you have done it before on some other matters. No one knows the hospital better than you."

Long grinned inwardly as he made these remarks, musing "No harm in feeding the ego." He thought, "If I can get Wood to take an active role, the medical staff activity almost certainly will result in Dr. Carter's promotion, and he will remain on the staff. Building Wood up as a power behind the scenes won't do any harm at all. I wonder whether Dr. Carter has talked to a lawyer yet? If he puts an attorney directly into the picture, lines will be drawn. I'll have less opportunity to manipulate Wood, and Wood will have less to manipulate people in the hospital."

The conversation ended with Wood saying he thought there might be "a few things" he could do.

* * * * *

Early the next day Wood met with Dr. Stanley Webb, a highly regarded internist on the staff whom he knew to be friendly with Dr. Carter and fairly well acquainted socially with a number of board members. Dr. Webb was a member of the Executive Committee of the medical staff and could be counted upon as a Carter ally. The administrator told Dr. Webb he feared that the Department of Orthopedics was going to make a negative recommendation on Dr. Carter's promotion and that he couldn't predict what the Executive Committee would do. Dr. Webb said he hadn't given it much thought but would be very disappointed if there was a negative departmental recommendation. He also said he would vote to recommend promotion, regardless of the department's position.

He explained that he had referred a number of cases to Dr. Carter over the last three years and believed his professional performance to be exemplary. He added that other staff members felt the same way. He believed a number of persons on the staff didn't think Drs. Archer and Baker had been "playing by the rules of the game" after Dr. Meyer's death and that Dr. Carter's willingness to help out the widow demonstrated he was a decent person.

Wood then asked Webb where the president of the staff, Dr. Martin Frank, would stand. Webb thought for a while, and then said:

"I think that Marty probably would vote to recommend Dr. Carter for promotion, regardless of what the people in orthopedics say. And he carries a lot of weight in the committee. However, I think you ought to know that most of the chairmen probably would take the view that they should defer to the recommendation of the department to which the physician is assigned, and it's my opinion that Dr. Carter will probably not get a positive recommendation from the Executive Committee if orthopedics votes against him. Personally, I would have no hesitation about talking to some of the people on the board to tell them, if the Executive Committee goes against Dr. Carter, that it is a lousy recommendation and that they shouldn't accept it."

After more conversation, the two parted.

* * * * *

At this point, Wood decided on the strategy he would follow if there was a negative recommendation from orthopedics. He reasoned that if the recommendation was positive, the Medical Staff Executive Committee would go along and, while Drs. Archer and Baker would be upset, the worst that could happen would be that they would shift more admissions to hospital X. That didn't worry him much. On the other hand, if orthopedics recommended against promoting Dr. Carter and the Executive Committee had to face the question of whether to overrule that decision, it was fairly likely to decline to do so, and the stage would be set for a hearing.

Then the selection of staff members for the hearing committee would be critical. Wood decided he would recommend to Dr. Frank, the staff president, that if orthopedics adopted a negative recommendation and the Executive Committee clearly was going to support it, that he refrain from voting. Dr. Frank then would appoint one member from each side in the Executive Committee and the staff president would make himself the third representative of that panel.

Wood also decided to meet with Benjamin Harris, the president of the hospital board and informally discuss the problem with him. The president then would understand the nature of the hospital's difficulty and this might have an effect on Harris's choices of the three members of the governing board to represent it on the hearing committee.

Wood then faced the question of whether he should confide in Long concerning his plan. He decided there was no particular advantage to doing so, reasoning that if the situation worked itself out as he hoped, there would not truly be a legal problem and the solution would be strictly in the realm of administration.

* * * * *

During the several days preceding the Orthopedics Department meeting, Dr. Carter spent a good deal time attempting to line up and maintain his support within the medical staff. He sought out opportunities to chat informally with several members of orthopedics to indicate his desire to remain on the staff, and he sought to allay concern about his behavior that might have arisen from remarks made by Drs. Archer and Baker about his performance and personal reliability.

He also sought to strengthen his contacts with members of other departments, and spoke at length with Dr. Webb, his friend who also was on the Executive Committee, and several other prominent physicians on the staff who had referred cases to him. From Dr. Webb and at least two other key physicians he received clear expressions of support and intimations that they would use their own influence with other members of the staff to maintain his appointment.

Drs. Archer and Baker were aware of Dr. Carter's politicking and were doing some themselves. Since all three spoke with physicians they assumed would be favorable to their own side, each of the protagonists felt the staff was largely behind him. Dr. Carter spoke with his attorney, Lewis, in the afternoon of the day of the department meeting. He told Lewis he felt things looked very good and believed he would get a favorable recommendation. The attorney replied that, while he was pleased that the situation seemed favorable, Dr. Carter should be prepared, at the minimum, if the recommendation was negative, to invoke the hearing procedure in the medical staff bylaws.

Lewis explained these procedures to Dr. Carter who, although associated with the hospital for his years of graduate training and for nearly three years on the medical staff, was unaware of them. Lewis asked whether Dr. Carter recalled any instances of neglect or questionable performance on his part that had been raised at departmental meetings or in any other hospital forum. Dr. Carter said he couldn't think of anything that would put him in a poor light. The conversation ended on a positive note, with Dr. Carter stating that he believed the situation would be resolved successfully at the departmental meeting. He planned to attend the session, at which recommendations for all members of the department were to be made, although he would have to leave the room while his case was discussed.

* * * * *

At the departmental meeting, all other business was completed rapidly. Dr. Robin, the chairman, decided that since Dr. Carter's recommendation was the only one that would raise conflict, it should be left for last. Only members of the active staff of the department were eligible to vote on recommendations. All other department members were rapidly approved for reappointment and continuation of their clinical privileges.

Dr. Robin then explained that Dr. Carter was at the point in the medical staff organization where a recommendation was necessary as to whether he be promoted to active staff or not be reappointed. Dr. Carter left the room and the meeting proceeded.

Dr. Archer made a statement in which he said he and Dr. Baker had been associated with Dr. Carter for nearly three years and had found numerous instances of carelessness in his work both at the hospital and in the office, and that he had neglected his duties by spending considerable time covering Dr. Meyer's practice after his death. He added that Dr. Carter, in violation of his contract, had sought and received payment for services to Dr. Meyer's patients and that his continued practice in the area and at the hospital was in violation of a covenant not to compete after leaving the employ of the partnership.

When he finished no one else sought to speak. A vote then was taken on Dr. Archer's motion to recommend that Dr. Carter not be advanced to the active staff. The tally—by secret ballot, at Dr. Robin's decision—was 4 to 2 in favor of a negative recommendation.

Dr. Carter was invited to return and informed that the department's negative recommendation would be sent the next day to the president of the staff for further consideration by the Medical Staff Executive Committee. As the meeting broke up, Dr. Carter was both disappointed and angry. On his way out of the building he was approached by Dr. Robert Fuller, a member of the Orthopedics Department, who sought to provide him with some solace. Dr. Fuller also said he had a few friends on the board and would contact them soon to let them know that, in his opinion, there was no basis to sustain the negative recommendation.

When Dr. Carter returned home he immediately called his attorney, Lewis, and they discussed the moves open to them. Lewis encouraged him to talk with as many staff members as he could who he thought were favorable to him and to suggest that if these allies had any leverage with the members of the Executive Committee or the board, they should not hesitate to use it on his behalf. Dr. Carter asked, "Is it ethical for me to get into this business in this way? I'm not running for election. All I'm doing is trying to stay on the staff of the hospital. The way I feel right now, I don't know whether I want to stay in a department that would treat me the way those people just did."

Lewis responded, "Forget about the vote tonight. That is all over with, and you and I know that you really want to and need to stay on the staff of the hospital. If you hadn't crossed Dr. Archer and Dr. Baker, all of those people would be your friends. What we have to do is make sure that the final decision is to promote you. Even if we lose with the board, we can always go to court."

Carter told his attorney about his short conversation with Dr. Fuller. Lewis said that the fact that Dr. Fuller had offered to assist augured well and that "you have only lost a skirmish, we are not even on the main battlefield yet."

* * * * *

The following day, Friday, after Wood, the administrator, learned of the Orthopedics Department vote, he found an opportunity to meet with Dr. Frank, the president of the staff. They discussed the Carter situation and Wood laid out his plan for handling it in the Executive Committee. Dr. Frank was noticeably disturbed by the negative recommendation, declaring:

"This is the first time since I've been on the Executive Committee, and I have been on it for the past four years, and was on it earlier for two years, that we ever had a negative recommendation about a member of the staff. Now, I know some people decided not to apply for reappointment and I know we have had a few instances where people were put under some special monitoring, but this is the first time we had a situation where the Executive Committee is going to have to vote up or down on a department recommendation to deny reappointment."

Wood said he didn't believe personalities should govern medical staff appointments. He commented that if Dr. Frank followed the approach he proposed, with either a positive or negative Executive Committee recommendation on Carter, the matter would be out of the hands of the medical staff, and the staff president's final step would be to appoint the members of the hearing committee. Wood ended by saying:

"Let things happen the way they will. Just remember that the board is not going to be very keen about deciding to refuse to keep Dr. Carter on the staff if the members think he might take the hospital to court. If you can find a way to help us prevent that eventuality, everyone will be better off."

Wood then met with Long, the hospital's attorney, at his office. The administrator described the decision and his conversation with Dr. Frank. Long commented:

"I think you've got a pretty good idea of how to handle this administratively. We have never had a hearing under these bylaws, and there may be some question with respect to how fair the procedure is. What I will do in the next few days is put on paper some of my thoughts on how the hearing should be conducted.

"Of course, if the Executive Committee votes to recommend Dr. Carter's advancement to the active staff, we won't need a hearing and we probably will have laid this matter to rest. I think that you had better be careful because, if Dr. Archer and Dr. Baker have a lot more friends on the staff than you believe they have, you are going to be in a difficult position if it appears that you have been taking sides."

Wood then asked Long to prepare a memorandum on the specific question of whether the hospital had any obligation to make a negative decision on a medical staff appointment because the physician was practicing contrary to a covenant not to compete in a contract with another physician. Long agreed and asked the administrator what he proposed to do with the memorandum. Wood replied, "I would like to show it to Dr. Frank and to anyone else on the medical staff or board who might inquire about what, if anything, the hospital's responsibility is in such a situation."

Long asked Wood whether he would attend the Executive Committee meeting. Wood said he would. The attorney then instructed him not to volunteer anything about the memorandum unless the issue was raised specifically by a member of the committee during its deliberations. Wood agreed he would not.

Many telephone calls were made over the weekend by Drs. Archer, Baker, and Carter and other members of the medical staff to members of the Executive Committee and some board members. Dr. Carter was cheered by the favorable reactions he received. A number of medical staff members called him to let him know they were either working on his behalf or at least sympathetic to his position and wished him well.

* * * * *

When the Executive Committee met at noon on Tuesday, for the first time as far as anyone could remember every member was present. All business, except for the Orthopedics Department recommendations, was concluded rapidly. The orthopedics recommendations then were brought up and all except Dr. Carter's were concurred with quickly.

The recommendation to not promote Dr. Carter to active staff was then before the committee. Dr. Frank, in the chair as staff president, explained briefly that a similar recommendation by the Executive Committee would entitle Dr. Carter to a hearing under the bylaws. He said a decision not to promote Dr. Carter would be the same as one to deny reappointment because of a provision in the medical staff bylaws that a physician was required to advance to the active staff from the associate staff within three years after obtaining membership.

Dr. Frank then asked Dr. Robin, the orthopedics chairman, to provide any information he believed useful to the Executive Committee. Dr. Robin stated briefly that Dr. Carter had been a member of orthopedics for three years, that all members of the department had had an opportunity to observe his performance, and that a majority had voted to recommend that he not be advanced to the active staff. One member of the Executive Committee asked, "Has there ever been such a situation presented to us before?"

"As far as I know, there has never been a formal negative recommendation of this kind," Dr. Frank replied, "but some doctors have left the staff under a cloud for reasons possibly related to their competence or their behavior. If these doctors had not withdrawn from further consideration, they almost certainly would have been given adverse recommendations."

Dr. Webb, the internist who was a member of the Executive Committee, asked to speak. He said, "I have closely followed Dr. Carter's work here. He has taken carc of patients I referred to him, and my associates referred to him, and his work has always been exceptionally good. Others on the staff have had similar good experiences."

He also referred to the fact that Dr. Carter had been in residency at the hospital and that no question had been raised about his performance during that period.

Dr. William Richards, chairman of the Pediatrics Department, then took the floor. He said he had only slight knowledge of Dr. Carter personally but felt a major principle was at stake.

"We have a large medical staff at this hospital, and for organizational purposes, it is divided into departments," Dr. Richards commented. "As individual members of the Executive Committee, we must rely on the evaluation made by members of the department to which a doctor is assigned, because they have the greatest opportunity to observe and to assess the performance of physicians within their department.

"Therefore, I am in favor of the Executive Committee's recommending that Dr. Carter not be promoted to the active staff because I have faith in the judgments made by his colleagues in orthopedics. If we cannot trust our brethren and the decisions they make, there is little reason to bother with obtaining recommendations from any departments in the hospital. There is a matter of principle at stake here, and I think that it cannot be overlooked."

Several other committee members then commented. Those who spoke in favor of the Executive Committee's upholding the Orthopedics Department emphasized that their position was based on the principle Dr. Richards had stated. Those who spoke in favor of a positive recommendation for Dr. Carter focused on the fact that orthopedics had provided no information as to the basis for its negative recommendation and pointed out that only the vote of the department, for reasons that were not stated specifically, was before them.

After 15 minutes of discussion, Dr. Frank, the staff president, called for a vote. The Executive Committee was composed of the officers of the staff, those who chaired the departments, and three members of the staff elected at large. The total membership was 15, of whom 9 were department heads. Dr. Frank asked whether the committee wanted to vote secretly or by a show of hands. There was no immediate response so he said that, unless he heard any objections, the vote would be by show of hands. He then stated the issue as follows:

"The question upon which we have to vote is whether to recommend to the board of the hospital that Dr. Carter not be promoted to the active staff, which will mean that if the board accepts our recommendation, the effect will be that his staff membership will be terminated as of the end of his current appointment."

Dr. Frank asked for a show of hands by those in favor of a negative recommendation, and seven of the nine department heads and one other member of the staff voted. When asked for a show of hands of those opposed to this recommendation, four members voted. Two committee members did not raise their hands either time, and Dr. Frank did not participate in the vote.

* * * * *

Within an hour, the result of the vote was known throughout the hospital. When Dr. Carter learned of it, he immediately called his attorney. Lewis asked whether he was prepared to request the hearing to which he was entitled under the medical staff bylaws. The young orthopedic surgeon said he was deeply offended by what had happened and was "ready to go all the way."

Lewis said Dr. Carter had 10 days after receipt of written notice of the negative recommendation to request a hearing, but that there was nothing to prevent him from doing so earlier. Lewis advised him to see Wood, the administrator, promptly to request a hearing orally and to announce that he would submit a letter within a day or so containing the formal request.

Wood, who had been silent throughout the Executive Committee meeting, telephoned the hospital attorney, Long, as soon as he returned to his office. As Wood described the session, his tone of voice betrayed concern. Long allowed him to finish, then said:

"This was not unexpected. We already have a plan for the next stage of this business. We expect that Dr. Carter will request a hearing, and the hospital will arrange for it to be held as promptly as possible. If you like, I will talk with the board president and advise him that under the bylaws he must now appoint three members of the board to serve on the hearing committee. Don't worry, he will get the picture, and he'll make appropriate choices.

"You should alert Dr. Frank that as president of the medical staff, he will have to choose three staff members from the Executive Committee, and he already should know how to make his selections. Make certain that he understands that someone on the Executive Committee should be prepared to present the case supporting the negative recommendation about Dr. Carter and that this person will have to present some kind of evidence to support the vote that was taken.''

''I can't picture what anyone apart from Dr. Archer and Dr. Baker can say that would lay any basis for the negative recommendation,'' Wood said. ''If nothing specific was brought up at the Executive Committee, how in the world will there be any specifics to bring to the hearing?''

''That is not your problem,'' Long replied. ''You just make sure that the hearing is scheduled and that Dr. Frank knows his responsibilities. The situation would be entirely different if someone really had something on Dr. Carter. But we will have to play out the script according to the bylaws and that is all there is to it.''

* * * * *

The next day Long called Benjamin Harris, president of the hospital board. After an exchange of conversational pleasantries, the hospital attorney described the nature of Harris's responsibilities at that point:

''Dr. Carter is entitled to a hearing and we are quite certain that he will request one. You must appoint three members of the board to serve on the hearing committee. They will be serving in a judicial role. They, along with three members of the Medical Staff Executive Committee, will then make a recommendation to the board on the question of whether you should accept the recommendation of the Executive Committee. The hearing committee may recommend that the board take the action recommended, or take other action appropriate to the circumstances and evidence brought forward at the hearing.

''It is my opinion that the board has an interest in avoiding litigation that probably would follow a decision adverse to Dr. Carter. To be upheld in the courts, I advise you that it would be necessary for the hospital to show that there was a basis for the adverse decision, based on evidence of poor professional performance, bad deportment, or something else that would make the action seem reasonable.''

''I have already received a telephone call about Dr. Carter, and I know that some of the other board members have received calls as well,'' Harris replied. ''We have never had such a situation at the hospital before, and I certainly don't want to be the first to get our medical staff business into court. How do you suggest that I choose members of the board for the hearing committee?''

Long responded, ''Why don't you pick from among members who have shown the greatest interest in the hospital, the ones who attend board meetings and do the committee work? Also, give some thought to whether they can adopt a judicial attitude. I don't believe I should mention any names to you. You know the members of the board better than I do anyway.''

''Suppose one or more of the people I pick has already received calls about the Carter situation, can I appoint any of them to serve on the hearing committee?'' Harris asked.

Long was prepared for that question and hesitated only briefly before saying, "I wouldn't worry about the fact that a board member has received a telephone call. When you contact a board member and he or she already has decided how to vote, you know that individual should not be appointed. Don't hesitate to call me if, when you approach a board member to serve, the person's reaction gives you some concern about possible bias. That's the kind of advice you pay me for."

Harris ended the conversation by commenting wryly, "Why didn't this wait until next year when I won't be president."

Long telephoned Wood to inform the hospital administrator of his conversation with Harris. He also directed Wood to send a letter to Dr. Carter advising him of the recommendation of the Executive Committee and informing him of his right to request a hearing. He told Wood not to mention anything in the letter about Dr. Carter's being permitted to have an attorney with him at the hearing. Long explained that the bylaws were silent on such representation but that if the physician later were to request this, specifically, Long would deal with the question at that time. He inquired whether Wood had talked yet with Frank.

"I spoke with Marty Frank early this morning," the administrator said. "I told him of his responsibility as staff president to appoint the members of the hearing committee, and to assign the responsibility for presenting the negative recommendation and any supporting materials to that group. Dr. Frank is very upset. He doesn't see much difficulty in selecting members of the hearing committee. He will appoint himself and, if they will serve, the two members of the Executive Committee who also abstained from voting on the recommendation at the meeting.

"I asked him whether he wanted to select one of the people who voted in favor of the negative recommendation and one who voted against, but he said he would prefer those who had abstained. He is not that concerned about the hearing committee. His problem is that he doesn't think he can find anyone to take the responsibility of presenting evidence against Dr. Carter. He approached Dr. Robin, the orthopedics chairman, who voted in favor of the negative recommendation in the Executive Committee, but Dr. Robin said he was unwilling to take the lead. Perhaps you had better talk with Dr. Robin and settle him down. I would not want to be in Dr. Robin's shoes right now."

"I think I can give Dr. Robin a way to handle the situation," Long said. "Do you think Dr. Frank will mind if I talk to Dr. Robin directly or do you think he should have Dr. Robin call me?"

"I don't think that Dr. Frank would have any objection," Wood replied. "Let me talk to him and I will get back to you."

Later that day Wood spoke with Dr. Frank, who said he would be happy to have Long talk with Dr. Robin. Wood called Long and told him the road was cleared for him to deal directly with Dr. Robin.

The hospital attorney then called Dr. Robin and said:

"As the chairman of the Orthopedics Department, you are the physician who should represent the Medical Staff Executive Committee before the hearing committee. Your responsibility is to put forward whatever information you or others have that concerns the qualifications, or the lack of them, for Dr. Carter's promotion to the active staff."

"I don't know what I can say that is bad about Dr. Carter," Dr. Robin responded. "I didn't vote on the department recommendation and the only reason I voted for the negative recommendation in the Executive Committee was that I felt that I should go along with the decision made within my department. I have nothing to say apart from reporting the results of the votes."

"That is not going to be particularly impressive to a hearing committee," the attorney said. "Why don't you contact Dr. Archer and Dr. Baker and tell them that, since they spoke so eloquently against Dr. Carter at the departmental meeting, they can make a return appearance and do their act again at a hearing?"

"But what if neither one is willing to come before the hearing committee?" Dr. Robin asked.

"I guess it will be a very short hearing," Long said.

"That would make the Executive Committee look pretty stupid. The board members will really wonder how we go about things in the medical staff," Dr. Robin complained.

"Perhaps a lesson will be learned if that happens," Long said. "This may turn out to be an educational experience for a lot of people."

Dr. Robin said he would go along with the scenario based on this conversation, adding, "I feel like I've been used."

Long telephoned Wood and reported his conversation with Dr. Robin. The administrator asked whether Long would be willing to meet with members of the hearing committee when it was appointed to describe the procedures that would be followed. Long said he would and that everything seemed in place for a hearing, assuming Dr. Carter submitted his request.

* * * * *

Disregarding his own attorney's advice, Dr. Carter did not visit Wood to request a hearing in person. He waited until the administrator's letter reached him, then met with Lewis at his office. The attorney described what he felt would be the next step based on the medical staff bylaws. He dictated a letter for Dr. Carter to sign requesting a hearing and seeking a statement of particular cases and instances of conduct that constituted the foundation for the negative recommendation. The letter also included a request for the presence of his attorney at the hearing, and for the hospital to inform him of the names of the members of the hearing committee at least five days before the session so he could prepare possible objections to the composition of the panel on the grounds of bias or lack of objectivity.

Lewis then asked which members of the medical staff Dr. Carter would want to testify as witnesses on his behalf. Lewis suggested that at least one be a member of a department other than orthopedics who could indicate satisfaction with his professional performance on the basis of cases referred to Dr. Carter. He recommended that the young surgeon select one member of the Orthopedics Department who could review, on his behalf, any specific cases that were mentioned as indicative of poor professional performance. This physician also would be able to testify with regard to his knowledge and evaluation of Dr. Carter's work in orthopedics during the preceding three years.

Dr. Carter mentioned both Dr. Stanley Webb, the member of the Medical Staff Executive Committee who had been very friendly, and Dr. Robert Fuller, the member of the Orthopedics Department who had been one of the two who voted against the negative recommendation. Lewis said they would be excellent witnesses and he would plan to meet with both.

Lewis explained that if the hospital denied the request for an attorney, they would then have to deal with the question of whether Dr. Carter should obtain another member of the medical staff to serve as his advocate. Lewis expressed the opinion that, if it became clear that a physician was going to present the case in favor of the negative recommendation, another physician, rather than Lewis, should serve as the Carter spokesman.

Dr. Carter said he was uncomfortable about being in a hearing without Lewis. The attorney assured him that he would devote sufficient time to instructing the physician who would be Dr. Carter's representative so he should not be apprehensive. "If I am in there to represent you, and a physician is on the other side, the physician will be able to get some sympathy regardless of how badly he performs, and my presence may actually be detrimental to your case," Lewis explained. "I have not talked with the hospital's attorney but, once the hearing is scheduled, I will get in touch with him and run over the ground rules. While I don't know Harry Long personally, by reputation I know him to be competent and hardworking and I don't think we will have any difficulty in establishing procedures that will give you adequate protection."

"Listen, to you this is just another case; for me it is maintaining my practice in this town," Dr. Carter exploded. "If I get knocked out of this hospital, even if I can get connected somewhere else, it is going to cost me a lot of money. If we decide to sue them if we don't win in the hospital, it also is going to be a lot of dollars."

"You are just like most clients," Lewis said soothingly. "I can't guarantee results. I'm just like a doctor. I'll do my best and I'm confident that you, or we—if you like that better—are in good shape. I want you to be getting the sympathy at the hearing, not some doctors I can make fools of. Unless they come up with some specific patients you killed or paralyzed by lousy practice, you should come out all right. If it goes the way I believe it will, you might pick up a couple of board members as patients."

"That is not very funny," Dr. Carter said tartly.

"I'm sorry." After a pause Lewis asked, "Is there anything that came up in the department meeting about your activities, deportment, or anything else, that might surface at the hearing?"

"Well, Dr. Archer talked about my contract with the partnership and said I was violating it," Dr. Carter said.

"What contract is that? You haven't told me about any contract." Long clearly was agitated.

"Oh! Well, when I joined Dr. Archer and Dr. Baker I signed a contract. Frankly, I don't know what was in it. They say now I am competing with them in violation of the agreement."

"I better take a look at the contract. Can you send me a copy?"

"I'm afraid I can't," Dr. Carter said. "I don't have a copy of it now. In fact, I don't think I ever received a copy."

"Did any lawyer review it for you before you signed?" Lewis asked.

"No, it seemed to be a formality. The only part I noticed was the amount of the salary. How important is it?"

"Without knowing what is in the contract, I can't tell you much," Lewis replied. "But, if they think you are in breach of contract, they should go to court, not try to get the hospital to punish you for that. After all, the contract has nothing to do with the hospital. Let me see what I can find out. Try to be more careful about contracts in the future. At least get a copy of anything you sign, if you don't get some legal advice first. Don't they teach you anything about contracts in medical school?"

* * * * *

Two days later the letter Lewis drafted for Dr. Carter reached Wood at the hospital. The administrator called Long and read the letter to him. Long then remarked, "Obviously Dr. Carter has an attorney now. Why don't you ask him who his attorney is and then I will deal directly with him in the procedural matters."

Long told Wood he would provide further instructions about the response to the letter and would make the most of the arrangements, attorney to attorney.

Wood was relieved to have Long take a more active role. He telephoned Dr. Carter and asked whether he had an attorney. The physician said he did and gave Chris Lewis's name. Wood explained that the hospital's attorney preferred to deal directly with his lawyer. Dr. Carter said that would be fine with him because he wanted to concentrate on practicing medicine.

When Long learned who represented Dr. Carter, he telephoned Lewis and they agreed to meet to discuss procedures relating to the hearing. At the meeting Long told Lewis that Dr. Carter or he would receive a letter indicating the specific matters to be presented to the hearing committee, as well as the names of the panel members, far enough in advance of the session so the physician would have an opportunity to raise questions about the group's composition. The two attorneys agreed on a date for the hearing two weeks later, dependent upon the availability of the committee members and expected witnesses.

The question of Dr. Carter's being represented by counsel at the hearing was then raised. The hospital attorney told Lewis, "My position is that the matter should be considered without your presence. A physician will be presenting the case against Dr. Carter, who can be represented by another member of the medical staff, or he can present his side on his own."

Lewis asked, "Will you be at the hearing?"

Long replied, "I'll be there solely to advise the hearing committee on procedures and whether it can consider items of evidence. I won't present evidence and I won't talk about the merits."

"I'll buy that," Lewis said. "We'll withdraw the request for legal representation. Perhaps we'll have another doctor accompany Dr. Carter, at least to hold his hand."

As the final matter in their discussion, Lewis asked Long what he felt the evidentiary burden was at the hearing, since the bylaws were silent on the matter. The hospital attorney said this was a question that concerned him and that it was unfortunate the bylaws said nothing. He proposed that the test be that Dr. Carter disprove the charges that were the basis for the negative recommendation by substantial evidence. Lewis countered with the proposal that the test be that the charges be supported by substantial evidence. The two fenced for quite some time on the subject without final agreement.

Long pointed out that the final decision, in terms of advising the hearing committee, was his, and that while he understood Lewis's position, he didn't feel that the subject was one upon which the two necessarily had to agree.

"If your man loses and we end up in court, the judge will decide whether my instructions to the hearing committee were proper," Long concluded.

* * * * *

In the next few days the hearing committee was constituted. The medical staff representatives were Dr. Frank, the staff president, and the two other Executive Committee members who had abstained; plus Harris, the president of the board, and two other board members who served on its executive committee. The names were promptly made known to Lewis and Dr. Carter, who made no objection to any of the individuals.

Lewis telephoned Long because neither he nor Dr. Carter had received the statement of any specific cases or other matters on which the hearing would focus. Long said some kind of notice would be sent out. He then telephoned Wood to find out what, if anything, Dr. Robin, the orthopedics chairman, had prepared. Wood said Dr. Archer had provided him with no specific cases but that he would speak at the hearing on Dr. Carter's "unprofessional, incompetent, and unethical practice" during the three years. Long told the administrator that such a statement of charges, consisting only of conclusions and lacking reference to specific instances, would not lay the basis for negative action that, if challenged in court, could be sustained.

"What do you expect me to do?" Wood asked rhetorically. "Dr. Robin doesn't want to carry this any further, Dr. Archer won't give him any specific information, Dr. Baker is in Kenya on a safari, and I'm sick of the whole thing."

"Perhaps we haven't done as good a job as we might have in this situation," Long said. "In any event, the hearing is scheduled, I have talked with Dr. Carter's attorney, and they will be prepared. I will be at the hearing to advise the committee as to procedures and evidentiary and other legal issues. Do you want to attend?"

"I can't think of anything I'd rather avoid more but I guess I had better be there and observe," Wood said. He then asked the hospital attorney whether there was anything else he should do for the hearing.

Long told Wood to call his secretary, who would make arrangements for a court reporter to be present. He also told Wood he would prepare a letter to be sent to Lewis stating that no specific cases would be brought up.

When Lewis received the letter from Long with no specific charges or cases, he called Dr. Carter and described the contents. He then said, "I don't know exactly how to prepare for this hearing because I can't understand what is going to be said in support of the negative recommendation of the Executive Committee. But we have to be fully prepared for whatever comes up. I want you to arrange for me to meet with Dr. Webb and Dr. Fuller (the two supportive members of the Executive Committee) within the next few days so we can plan their testimony."

Dr. Carter agreed to set up a meeting for the Monday night preceding the hearing, which was scheduled for a Thursday evening. The meeting with Dr. Webb and Dr. Fuller was rather short. Lewis explained the peculiar situation he faced because of the absence of any specificity of charges. The physicians explained their views as to the basis of the negative recommendation. Both suggested that the reason there was no specificity was simply because there was no basis to decline to advance Dr. Carter to the active staff.

Lewis described the nature of the testimony he wanted Dr. Carter to elicit from Dr. Webb. Basically, Dr. Webb was to testify as to the high regard in which Dr. Carter was held by members of the medical staff generally and that his care of patients Dr. Webb had referred to him was exemplary. Dr. Webb said he could refer to some specific cases by number and would arrange to have several of the charts with him.

Dr. Fuller said he would testify based on his observation of Dr. Carter's work during his training and his time on the medical staff. He explained that he had been heavily involved with Dr. Carter during his training and had referred several of his cases to him because of conflicts in scheduling, vacation, and similar reasons. He said he would mention that he had always reviewed the care provided in these cases and had found it to be consistent with the quality of performance he expected from himself and other competent members of the active staff.

Lewis was very pleased that there would be this strong pro-Carter testimony. However, Dr. Carter was very unhappy with the idea that he would be presenting the case on his own behalf. He asked whether some other physician should be found to accompany him and ask the questions of Dr. Webb and Dr. Fuller. Lewis said they would discuss this later, and the two potential witnesses left.

Lewis explained that he didn't think it was necessary for Dr. Carter to be accompanied by anyone from the staff since he had such positive witnesses available. He then explained the hearing procedure, based on the medical staff bylaws and his discussion with Long.

The attorney said that if no specific charges were made about the care of individual patients and Dr. Archer merely rambled on about poor performance, bad deportment, etc., he should merely ask Dr. Archer to indicate specific instances. Lewis provided questions to ask if such instances were mentioned. He told Dr. Carter that if Dr. Archer mentioned the provisions of the contract, he should point out for the benefit of the hearing committee that he did not consider himself to be in breach of any contract and, in any event, it was not the business of the hospital, but rather of the courts, to enforce contracts between physicians that did not involve the institution.

Although Dr. Carter was apprehensive, he seemed more assured than he had been earlier. They agreed to meet again the night before the hearing to prepare an outline of how he would proceed. Lewis instructed Dr. Carter to bring with him a copy of his curriculum vitae.

* * * * *

When Dr. Carter arrived, he asked why Lewis wanted the curriculum vitae. Lewis said, "I didn't mention this before but you are going to make a statement at the hearing. Actually, you will be testifying on the record about your training and your accomplishments, and giving the hearing committee an opportunity to know you better. Let me see your c.v."

Dr. Carter handed it to Lewis, who scanned it quickly, then said:

"This is not too bad. I will revise it to put the material in what I consider the best order for presentation. We'll get this redone and back to you with at least 10 copies by early tomorrow afternoon. Before you have Dr. Webb and Dr. Fuller testify I want you to make a statement describing your background and professional activities in greater detail than you will have in the c.v. You will have enough copies to give to every member of the hearing committee, and a few extras for anybody else who wants one."

"You keep on adding to what I have to do," Dr. Carter complained. "First, you arrange it so that you would not be present at the hearing. Then you talk about me being assisted or represented by another member of the medical staff. Then you decide that I should do the whole thing myself. Now you are telling me that I am going to be a witness. I can't help it but I am starting to feel as if I will have to blame myself if I lose."

Lewis laughed.

"I can understand how you feel I have been stringing you along," he said. "Another lawyer might have done things differently. I want to make this as low-keyed and as professionally oriented as possible. I am not looking at the problem as one involving courtroom drama. The reason I want you to do as much as the plan calls for is that I want to establish, partly through your personal involvement, that you are not seeking to make this a legal dispute at this time but prefer to keep it within the hospital family. You need to give the impression that you are respected by your peers, except for a few who aren't very credible. Take a look at these lists."

Lewis handed Dr. Carter several pages of paper. They were headed "Questions to Ask Dr. Webb," "Questions to Ask Dr. Fuller," "Statement to Make If the Issue of the Covenant Not to Compete Is Raised," "Introductory Remarks," "Closing Statements," and "Objections." While Dr. Carter skimmed the pages Lewis explained:

"You don't have to commit these to memory. You can leave them right there on the table in front of you and read from them when necessary, deviate to some extent from them when you think it is appropriate, and ignore parts of them if it appears to you that that is the wise thing to do. I want you to impress Dr. Frank and the board members particularly that you feel you have been wronged already, that a further injustice may be perpetrated unless they decide in your favor, and that you are rightfully indignant."

The two spent another half-hour reviewing the material in detail. Lewis said he would be in and out of the office most of Thursday but that if Dr. Carter needed any last-minute assistance, he would make certain that he would be back in touch.

* * * * *

By the time all the members of the hearing committee appeared at the hospital board room, where the hearing was to take place, it was more than 15 minutes after the scheduled time of 7 P.M. Then came the introductions of the members of the committee to each other, to Dr. Robin, the orthopedics chairman, to Dr. Carter, and to Long, the hospital attorney. Harris, the board president, who had designated himself chairman of the hearing committee, began the session. He had before him a sheet provided by Long indicating the order in which the steps of the hearing were to take place, and handed copies to both Dr. Robin and Dr. Carter. After stating the purpose of the hearing, Harris called on Dr. Robin, who rose and said:

"I was appointed, and I assure you I did not seek this opportunity, to present the recommendation of the Executive Committee of the medical staff. The recommendation is that Dr. Carter not be advanced to the active staff. This is based on the recommendation not to advance Dr. Carter that we received from the Orthopedics Department."

As Dr. Robin spoke he scanned the room in vain for Dr. Archer, who had promised him that afternoon that he would be present and speak. Dr. Robin continued, "I was counting on Dr. Frank Archer of our Department of Orthopedics to testify at this point in the hearing. I do not see him here in the board room and I wonder whether you will permit me to telephone him and remind him that he is supposed to be here."

Harris asked Long what he thought should be done. Long told Harris to grant a 10-minute recess. Harris then said, "The hearing is recessed for 10 minutes so that Dr. Robin can try to reach Dr. Archer."

During the recess Dr. Robin had Dr. Archer paged in the hospital and called at both his home and office, all without success. He was able to reach only the answering service, which responded that "the doctor will get back to you, please leave your name and telephone number."

A very unhappy Dr. Robin returned to the board room and the hearing resumed. He said, "I have nothing more to say. Dr. Archer is not in the hospital, he is not at home, and I cannot reach him through his office. At this point I don't know what to do."

Harris, the board president, turned to Long, who said, "You, and the members of the hearing committee, can ask Dr. Robin any questions that you feel may elicit information that you need in order to make your decision. Dr. Robin, I am sure, will tell you what he can."

Harris asked whether any member of the hearing committee had any questions. One board member, Carlton Trask, asked, "Why was this recommendation made about Dr. Carter? Have we received any report stating the reasons for the Executive Committee's recommendation?''

''There is no report.'' Dr. Robin replied. ''I can't tell you exactly why any member of the Executive Committee voted in favor of this recommendation, against the recommendation, or'' and he looked straight at Dr. Frank, the staff president, ''why any doctor abstained from voting.''

The board member continued, ''You voted, didn't you?''

Dr. Robin responded, ''Yes, I did.''

''How did you vote?''

''I voted to recommend that Dr. Carter not be advanced to the active staff.''

''Why did you vote that way?'' Trask asked.

''Because the Orthopedics Department recommended that Dr. Carter not be advanced to the active staff.''

''Why did the Orthopedics Department vote the way it did?''

''I can't tell you why particular physicians voted one way or the other for certain,'' Dr. Robin responded.

The board member pressed on. ''Surely, there must be some reasons.''

''Well, if Dr. Archer were here, he could give some.''

''I can't understand why we are here if you don't have anything particular to say about Dr. Carter, and Dr. Archer isn't here,'' Trask said with obvious annoyance.

''You know I tried to reach Dr. Archer. That's about all I can do,'' Dr. Robin said apologetically.

Trask turned his attention to Harris and asked the board president:

''What is going on here? Can't we get any information from anybody?''

Long, the hospital attorney, spoke up:

''This is a hearing. This is not an investigation. I am surprised that Dr. Archer is not present but we might as well go ahead with the hearing.''

''Listen, Dr. Robin, we are not holding you responsible for Dr. Archer's absence,'' Harris said. ''However, I can't understand why we are here either.''

During the exchange between Trask, the board member, and Dr. Robin, Dr. Webb, the pro-Carter internist and member of the Executive Committee, struggled to maintain a straight face. He had talked with this board member that afternoon and had primed him to ask questions of Dr. Archer. Dr. Webb thought to himself that things were turning out perfectly for Dr. Carter.

Harris had a short conversation with Long, then asked Dr. Carter whether he had anything to say about the negative recommendation.

Dr. Carter began haltingly, glancing frequently at the papers Lewis had given him and some notes he had made. He held up a copy of his curriculum vitae and said he wanted to introduce it as evidence. He then handed out copies to all hearing committee members. He waited while they glanced at it, then said, ''I could amplify what is there but I think the best thing for me to do is to answer any questions you have about the content of my c.v.''

Harris asked, ''You trained here, didn't you?''

''That is right there on the c.v.,'' Carter responded. ''I did all my orthopedic training here and I finished in 1969.''

No one else on the committee had any questions and Dr. Carter, feeling more confident as he went along, then called Dr. Webb to testify. Following the list of questions that Lewis had prepared, Dr. Carter elicited the expected favorable remarks. After Dr. Webb finished, Harris asked Dr. Robin whether he had any questions. The orthopedics chairman said he did not. Harris then asked the hearing committee members whether they had any questions. They declined to ask any.

Dr. Carter then introduced Dr. Fuller, one of his supporters in orthopedics, who gave the expected answers to questions regarding Dr. Carter's performance as an orthopedist. When he finished, Dr. Robin was given the opportunity to ask questions, which he declined.

Dr. Frank, the staff president, then asked, ''Do you think Dr. Carter is qualified to be an orthopedist on the active staff of this hospital?''

''I certainly do.'' Dr. Fuller responded. ''If I didn't think he was, I wouldn't be here. If Frank Archer truly thought Dr. Carter should not be on the staff here as an orthopedist, Dr. Archer would be here.''

Long instructed the members of the hearing committee to disregard the remark about Dr. Archer. Harris then asked whether there was anything anyone wanted to say or to ask. Otherwise, he said, the hearing would be closed.

Silence reigned. Harris declared the hearing concluded. It was only an hour after it had begun, and 10 minutes of the time had been devoted to a recess. The board president asked Long what to do next. The attorney suggested that the hearing committee members discuss what they would recommend to the hospital board. Long said he would sit in with them but he had no vote and he would not give an opinion as to the course they should take. He told them he was there strictly as an adviser on the procedures.

* * * * *

After the board room was cleared of everyone except the members of the hearing committee and Long, Harris asked the attorney:

''What do we have to give the board? We didn't get anything except a recommendation from the Executive Committee in writing. I think we need to have some kind of statement to submit to the board.''

''First, discuss the recommendations you might make,'' Long replied. ''Then, take a poll to decide whether you want to recommend that Dr. Carter be advanced to the active staff or whether you want to recommend that he not be advanced. After you decide that, we can discuss what should be in the statement to go to the board along with the recommendation.''

Harris immediately asked the other committee members whether any were interested in recommending that Dr. Carter not be advanced to the active staff. No one responded. Harris then said:

''I take it that we will recommend that Dr. Carter be advanced. I think our statement should say that there is no reason based on Dr. Carter's professional performance or conduct for not advancing him. Besides, two highly regarded staff members have given us their opinions that he is a competent surgeon and qualified for the active staff. Really, without any evidence about Dr. Carter that would lead to doubts about him, there is no basis for an adverse recommendation.''

He turned to Long and asked, ''Do we have to wait until we see the transcript of the testimony before we make our recommendation?''

''No,'' Long said. ''I can draft a statement based on what you have said and send the draft to all of you to approve before making it final. However, I'd like to see a formal vote on a motion to recommend that Dr. Carter be advanced.''

Harris asked for a motion to recommend that Dr. Carter be advanced to the active staff, and one of the board members made it. It was seconded promptly, then approved unanimously. Long again agreed to prepare the draft and distribute it promptly for comment and approval and the meeting of the hearing committee broke up.

Dr. Carter quickly called Lewis at home and described what had occurred. He was elated, almost jubilant, and Lewis attempted to calm him down.

''Do you know when the hearing committee will give its report to the board?'' Lewis asked.

''Nothing was said about that at the hearing and I didn't think to ask anyone.''

''Well, there still may be some kind of hitch, although I am quite confident the board will advance you to the active staff,'' Long said. ''You see, the board has already held its June meeting and unless it calls a special meeting, it will not be able to consider the report of the hearing committee until its next session, which will be in July, after your current appointment has expired. Tomorrow morning I will contact the hospital's attorney and have him make some arrangement so you can continue your appointment until there is a final determination by the board. I don't think this will be difficult to accomplish but I don't want you to have any difficulties that we can eliminate by prompt action now.''

''I am looking forward to seeing Dr. Archer and Dr. Baker around the hospital now,'' Dr. Carter said. ''For weeks I have been avoiding them and it is about time for them to start avoiding me.''

"While you are in such a good mood, let me ask you a question. Since you think everything went so well at the hearing, do you think it would have gone better, or worse, if I had been there representing you?"

"I don't know and I don't care. You will have to excuse me now. I have some more people to call to tell them about the hearing."

* * * * *

The next day Lewis and Long conferred about the gap between the end of Dr. Carter's present appointment and the time the board would meet to consider the hearing committee report. After reviewing the medical staff bylaws, Long said he would arrange for Dr. Robin, the chairman of orthopedics, to grant temporary privileges to Dr. Carter, if that were necessary, to cover the period until the board meeting. This was agreeable to Lewis and he promptly told Dr. Carter how that problem would be solved.

During the next two weeks the hearing committee report was drafted, circulated, and approved unanimously by all members. It recommended that Dr. Carter be advanced to the active staff of the hospital. A copy was provided to Lewis.

At the July board meeting, the recommendation of the Medical Staff Executive Committee and the report and recommendation of the hearing committee were presented. After a brief discussion, prompted by several questions to Harris about the conflict between the recommendations, the board voted to appoint Dr. Carter to the active staff. Wood, the administrator, promptly informed him of this decision.

* * * * *

Four years later the situation was as follows:

Dr. Carter had a heavy volume orthopedic practice at hospital Y in association with two other orthopedists he had recruited to join him; Dr. Archer and Dr. Baker no longer were on the staff of hospital Y, having shifted their practice to hospital X; and hardly anyone recalled that there had been a question about Dr. Carter's continuing at hospital Y.

Commentary

1.

It might very well be asked why, once it became apparent to Wood and Long that there was no substantive basis for denying Dr. Carter's advancement to the active staff, they failed to influence the process of consideration of his status and attempt to avoid the need for a hearing. As administrator, Wood might have taken a more active role, once the Orthopedics Department recommendation was made, to explain to the Executive Committee what was required for a recommendation adverse to Dr. Carter that would be sustained by the board and, if challenged further, by a court.

If Wood were uncertain, he could have sought counsel from Long, the hospital attorney. Long had become involved well before the Executive Committee meeting on the Carter recommendation. He could have initiated an informational session with some, or all, of the members to discuss the legal situation the hospital would be placed in if there was a negative recommendation that was not substantiated by evidence that would provide a basis for failing to advance him to the active staff. With more forceful intervention by Wood and/or Long, a negative recommendation might well have been avoided entirely and the need for a hearing eliminated.

The role of the hospital attorney is not always made very clear to the lawyer or well understood by the administration, medical staff, and board. Although the hospital is perceived to be a single institution, which it is under the law, at different times one or another of its elements may be in particular need of legal guidance. On occasion, different elements within the hospital may have conflicting views, or adverse positions, on specific matters, and one or more may desire or solicit the views of the attorney on the question at hand.

For example, the administration may seek advice as to its responsibility or authority on a particular matter when the medical staff has a different view of that power. The medical staff leadership also may seek the attorney's advice on the same matter, or at least desire it. It may become necessary for the hospital attorney to recommend that another lawyer, unconnected with his office, provide advice in such circumstances because he perceives he faces a conflict of interest.

The problem of conflict is manifest in the disciplinary setting. If the hospital attorney assists the medical staff in preparing and presenting charges against a member, that same lawyer cannot advise a hearing panel concerning the charges, procedural, and evidentiary matters at the hearing, and/or advise the governing board in its review of, and in making its final decision on, the recommendation of a hearing panel, without raising serious due process problems.

In the case study, the Executive Committee (the designated leadership group for the medical staff) was entitled to receive legal advice as to its recommendation role and the possible effects of its decisions. At minimum, Long could have offered to discuss with the panel the law relating to medical staff appointment and reappointment in the state, to enable the members to understand better the ramifications of any actions they decided to take.

It might be assumed that in this instance, Long would have explained that in the absence of any specific instances of poor professional performance or conduct rising to the level of cause for termination of an appointment, a decision based on a recommendation not supported by evidence of such failings would be likely to be overturned in court. That might well have given pause to the Executive Committee members who voted to support the principle that they must endorse a departmental recommendation.

2.

Dr. Carter's attorney decided he would not appear at the hearing on his client's behalf. Lewis chose this course after learning that there were no specific bases arising from Dr. Carter's professional performance or conduct upon which the negative recommendation was reached. The absence of specific allegations before the hearing meant that if any were to be raised at the session, Dr. Carter would have been in a strong position to assert in a subsequent court proceeding that he had been denied procedural due process. While the presence of counsel would not have eliminated that opportunity, Dr. Carter's attorney may have believed that his client's position would be even stronger if he had not had a lawyer present when such a departure from due process occurred.

The assessment that the hearing committee might be more sympathetic to Dr. Carter if he appeared without counsel may have been sound, too. While it is difficult to gauge the impact an attorney's presence may have on a hearing panel of physicians and board members serving in an adjudicatory role, in some situations it may be beneficial to the medical staff member to give the impression that counsel is not needed because what is "right" is so clear.

3.

At several points in the case study, the issue of the content and effect of the contract between Dr. Archer and Dr. Baker on the one hand, and Dr. Carter on the other, was raised. The advice given concerning the contract was sound.

Covenants not to compete are enforceable to at least some extent under state law and frequently are included in physician agreements.

The issue of the contract never was directly placed before either the executive or hearing committees and, as the case study indicates, never was examined by attorneys for either the hospital or Dr. Carter.

The hospital was not a party to the contract. Therefore, it was in no way obligated to assist Drs. Archer and Baker in enforcing it even if the contract was explicit on where Dr. Carter could not practice. Physicians should pursue such disputes through the courts. The hospital is not an appropriate forum and should not be used in a private dispute. Even if Dr. Archer had produced a contract that the hospital attorney believed was ironclad, and that a court would have enforced to the extent of preventing Dr. Carter from continuing to practice in the area and at hospital Y, it still would not have been the hospital's responsibility to assist the partners by denying reappointment to Dr. Carter solely on that basis.

There are instances in which physicians have sought to involve hospitals in other private disputes. Physician A may contract with Physician B to have the latter take patient histories and perform physicals for A's patients at a set fee per individual. The hospital becomes involved when Physician B, who has contracted to do the work, stops doing it because he asserts that A is substantially in arrears in his payments.

The problem comes to light because of the absence of histories and physicals on patient charts. When the hospital seeks to enforce its requirement for proper maintenance of medical records, Physician A, whose patients' records are not complete, charges Physician B with breaking a contract, and states that B should be disciplined, not he.

This type of dispute is a private one between two physicians over compensation for work done. The ultimate responsibility for maintenance and completion of medical records is with the attending physician (A) and, while he may assign or delegate that responsibility within some limits to another physician (B), such action does not relieve him of the responsibility as far as the hospital is concerned.

4.

In many medical staff controversies, an attempt is made to bend the hospital to the will of a particular physician or group of doctors by a threat to withhold admissions so as to affect the occupancy rate adversely. In some instances this may be effective. Such conduct, or even organizing to implement such a threat, may give rise to a basis for the hospital to take legal action. Whenever physicians make such a threat or take such an action, the hospital attorney must become involved promptly. A legal response is available and, on occasion, the fact that the hospital contemplates such a step may itself bring about termination of the threat or action.

While a shift in admitting practices by an individual physician would not ordinarily give rise to a basis for legal action, doctors' concerted action to influence a decision by the hospital board might well do so. There are difficult matters of proof in such cases but the frequency of such threats suggests that it is an area in which the hospital attorney should be prepared. In the case study, the threat did not go beyond possible action by the partnership of Dr. Archer and Dr. Baker. However, if they had sought to involve other physicians, serious consideration of a legal response would have been appropriate.

Case 2

Oh, What Webs We Weave

PERSONAE

Fred Anderson, administrator of Riverside Hospital
Dr. Bernard Arnold, member of Credentials Committee
Mrs. Helen Bellows, head of Medical Records Department
Dr. Herman Brown, earlier complainant about Dr. Silver
Dr. Samuel Carver, cardiac surgeon
Dr. Roger Connors, orthopedic surgeon and chairman of Credentials Committee
Bud Davis, reporter, friend of Anderson
Dr. Francis DeGaugh, earlier complainant about Dr. Silver
Dr. Harry Ginsberg, chief cardiologist
Dr. William Grant, orthopedic surgeon, subject of lawsuits
Dr. Wilfred Harrison, member of Credentials Committee
Dr. George Hutchins, suspended in an earlier case
Dr. Fred Keaton, anesthesiologist
Sara Kirts, Medical Records staff person
Arnold Little, attorney for Riverside Hospital
Dr. Charles Perkins, member of Credentials Committee
Ronald Sampson, attorney for Dr. Silver
Dr. Harold Silver, anesthesiologist, protagonist
Dr. Theodore Smith, member of Credentials Committee
Dr. Lester Strong, cardiac surgeon and chief of staff of Riverside Hospital
Don Thomas, racquetball player with Arnold Little
Dr. Peter Williamson, medical staff member

Dr. Charlie Wilson, medical staff member

Dr. Ursula Wolfe, chief of anesthesiology who investigated Dr. Silver

Overhead the big cumulus clouds were building. It looked and smelled like rain. Bill Grant didn't care about the weather. What he cared about was lining up his birdie putt on the 18th green at the Riverside Country Club and the cool beer waiting in the clubhouse. The beer there would taste especially good when his regular Wednesday afternoon golf buddies paid off the $10 Nassau for the 71 he was about to push down their throats. His putt eased over the lip and into the cup.

Bill Grant was William F. Grant, M.D., a noted orthopedic surgeon in Riverside, the central city of a metropolitan area of more than one million people on the banks of the Mississippi River. Bill was 41, a great college athlete who had kept himself in good shape and played what he believed to be one of the best games of golf in Riverside. He was a great guy and had a booming medical practice.

Booming was a perfect description of Dr. Grant. The first words out of his mouth always got everyone's attention. Nobody missed his jokes because everyone listened. Everyone enjoyed listening to Dr. Grant and Dr. Grant enjoyed everyone's listening.

He was enjoying himself with his golf partners in the clubhouse and was laughing at Joe Williams's recounting the three-putt 12th green when an older gentleman in a business suit approached and asked, "Are you Dr. Grant, Dr. William F. Grant?"

"That's right!" Bill exclaimed. His reply seemed louder than necessary. Then, quietly, Bill asked, "What can I do for you?"

"Nothing," the stranger said. "Here," almost throwing several papers into Bill's lap.

The stranger obviously was uncomfortable in his business suit in the 85-degree temperature. Even in the air conditioned clubhouse he perspired. Maybe he just wasn't a golfer. He turned to leave as Dr. Grant picked up the papers. Again, in a booming voice, "Hey! Wait a minute!" Bill said. "What's this all about?"

"It's a lawsuit," the man said. "I don't read'em, I just serve'em."

"Well I'll be damned," Dr. Grant said as he went through the papers, not really reading any of them. He acted as if by reading he would get involved in something he wanted no part of. Lawyers use such long paper and he wasn't a lawyer, but he was involved and he knew why. Two names jumped out at him, Chinn and Silver.

"What a way to ruin a great day. Harold Silver has really got me this time. Look at this!" he exclaimed to Dr. Harry Ginsberg. "Remember the Chinn case where Dr. Silver starved the Chinn boy of oxygen while I was operating on his knee? It affected his motor control! Well, before the operation he was the star quarterback on the East Riverside High team and I was trying to fix his knee so he could play next year. Silver makes it so he can't even pick up a ball, let alone throw it. What a tragedy. We're lucky we didn't have a vegetable on our hands. So now his parents have sued me, and the mistakes of Dr. Silver—super anesthesiologist—are now my problems and the problems of Riverside Hospital. What a mess."

"Sorry to leave guys," Dr. Grant said, "but I don't want to wrestle with the top on my 450 SL. I think I'll get home before it rains."

"Hey! Wait a minute," Dr. Ginsberg said, pointing at the papers, "you forgot your present."

* * * * *

Those cumulus clouds were the leading edge of a warm front that had brought a steady rain, still falling the next morning when Dr. Lester Strong, chief of staff at Riverside Hospital, pulled into the doctors' parking lot and stepped out of his Rolls Royce. Even in the rain he could not help but look back at the 1976 Silver Cloud of which he was extremely proud. As he started running through the downpour toward the emergency room door, he heard his name being called in Dr. Grant's bold, vibrant voice:

"Hey Dr. Strong! Wait up a minute! We've got to solve a problem, and we've got to solve it now!"

"Come on, Bill," Dr. Strong said. "We can't solve it out here, it's too damn wet. Let's talk in the Doctors' Lounge."

"No way, Les. This is a matter that I don't want everyone to hear, and the walls have ears in this hospital. Let's sit in your car. I've always liked to look at mahogany dashboards. Besides, I like the smell of leather upholstery a hell of a lot better than the strong coffee stench in the Doctors' Lounge. I sure wish they could get some decent coffee at this joint."

"All right, Bill. But only 10 minutes. I've got to get on with my rounds. This is a hell of a way to start the day."

Dr. Grant never could figure out what Dr. Strong saw in Rolls Royces. They drove like tanks. Maybe the ride was better—quieter, anyway—but lousy gas mileage, no pickup, and they made you feel like a stuffed shirt. Oh, well, to each his own.

"Listen, Les. Something has got to be done about Harold Silver. He's going to kill somebody. Look at this."

Dr. Grant shoved the *Summons and Complaint,* soiled, wrinkled, and now slightly wet, into Dr. Strong's hands.

"It's a claim for $2.5 million and Dr. Silver has no insurance. Doesn't that leave the hospital and me in the old sitting duck's position? That was too bad about the Chinn boy and I feel sorry about it, too, but that isn't what I came to talk about. This is just one of the many episodes in the saga of Dr. Silver."

Outside, the rain covered the windows like a sheet, making the conversation seem especially private. Inside, Dr. Grant was talking about Dr. Harold Silver, an anesthesiologist from New York State who had taken his training in Boston and had moved to Riverside some 18 months ago. Dr. Silver had fouled up on a number of cases he had handled for doctors on the four staffs to which he was admitted in the Riverside area. Nobody was comfortable with his work but anesthesiologists were hard to come by, so every once in a while they had to resort to him. The topic of discussion in the '76 Silver Cloud on Thursday morning was the record of, or better, the rumors about, Dr. Silver.

Dr. Strong did not care for the idea of knowing the "secret" truth; besides, the "truth" was only rumors. He opened the car window about an inch and said, "O.K., Bill, I agree. I'll talk to Fred Anderson as soon as I finish my rounds and we'll try to figure out what we can do. You get hold of Ursula Wolfe and see if she will meet me in Anderson's office around a quarter after ten and please, contact your insurance carrier."

"O.K. See you later."

Both doors opened and closed simultaneously. The doctors raced to get out of the rain.

* * * * *

Fred Anderson, the hospital's administrator, was 50 years old and looked it. He was balding, overweight, and hated exercise. He got things done by having an excellent rapport with the medical staff, the nursing staff, and the employees of the hospital. He wasn't a great wit or a dynamic speaker who could sell his board by oratory at its monthly meetings. He was a doer who dogged a problem by one-on-one contact with the people involved. He hated confrontations and meetings involving members of the medical staff because they always seemed so disorganized. He detested anarchy, but here he was in his plush office in Riverside Hospital talking with the chief of staff, Dr. Lester Strong; the chief of anesthesiology, Dr. Ursula Wolfe; and one of the best orthopedic surgeons around, Dr. William Grant.

Anderson looked across the room at Dr. Wolfe and thought to himself, she was too good-looking to be a doctor—she made him wish he were 20 years younger. Or half a million dollars richer. Besides looks, she was a damned good anesthesiologist. He was mentally tracing the curve of her belly from her ribs to her thigh when she suddenly pulled her smock tightly about her.

"All right, doctors. What's on your minds?"

"Dr. Harold Silver!" Dr. Grant exclaimed. "We've gotta bounce him off the staff."

Anderson was relieved to have a spokesman for the group. "Listen, Bill," he said, "I've heard about the Chinn suit. It is a ticklish situation, but it hasn't even been tried. We were served just yesterday. We can't use that as the basis to remove him from the staff."

Dr. Grant had talked Anderson into suspending another doctor a year and a half ago under his authority as the administrator to summarily suspend a physician who is a danger to patients. Anderson recalled the administrative headaches that had caused him when the doctor appealed. The overly complicated medical staff procedures were patterned after guideline bylaws of the Joint Commission on Accreditation of Hospitals. He had felt helpless waiting for the seemingly endless hearings to end before a resolution was reached. He felt even worse when he lost. He wasn't about to get into that administrative hassle again.

The procedures were good, you just could not count on the results. On this, Anderson and Dr. Wolfe were in agreement. She had served on the Review Committee on the case of Dr. George Hutchins, the one Anderson was recalling. She also had had her stomach full of late-night meetings, mostly with Dr. Hutchins's attorney. Talk about due process!

She was more intent now on streamlining the bylaws than she was on joining Dr. Grant's crusade, although she did agree that Dr. Silver wasn't much of an anesthesiologist.

Dr. Strong sucked on his pure briar pipe and joined Anderson in questioning Dr. Grant as to why Dr. Silver should be removed from the staff.

"Come on Bill," he said, "put your facts on the table and remember the Chinn case isn't part of the deck, at least not right now."

"Look," Dr. Grant exclaimed, "we all know that this guy is a lousy anesthesiologist and shouldn't be on our staff, so let's do something about it."

Anderson declared that, "I'm not doing anything without facts. If you've got a complaint, let's get it out on the table and see if it has enough merit to submit to the Credentials Committee."

"Well, Fred," Dr. Grant said, "I made a list of those cases that I have heard Dr. Silver has botched in the last 18 months. I suggest we give a copy to Dr. Wolfe and have her check them out, since Dr. Silver is in her department."

Everyone was anxious to see the list, and after reviewing it all realized there was more than smoke to Dr. Grant's accusations. It was agreed that Dr. Wolfe would check out the cases and report back to Anderson and Dr. Strong. As she started to leave, Anderson smiled and said, "If there is anything I can do to help you, Dr. Wolfe, please let me know."

* * * * *

Dr. Wolfe decided to go to the Doctors' Lounge to look for Dr. Charlie Wilson, the medical staff gossip. What better way to start an investigation of sour cases of which the souring ingredient was Dr. Silver. As she left the administrative area she took up a more purposeful stride down the long hall past the pharmacy and physical therapy to climb the stairs to the Doctors' Lounge on the second floor of the surgical wing. As she entered the lounge the smell of stale cigarette smoke invaded her nostrils, causing her to say out loud to no one in particular, "Why in the hell don't doctors practice what they preach. They blame their lack of willpower on the pressures of the medical world." She looked around the lounge but didn't see Dr. Wilson.

"Hey, Pete!" she cried.

Dr. Peter Willamson turned, concealing his cigarette, and gave her his best smile. "Yes, Dr. Wolfe?"

"Have you seen Charlie Wilson?"

"Is there a reward?"

"No funny stuff. I've got to pick his brain to start an investigation I've been assigned."

"Yeah? What's it all about?"

"Can't tell you right now. Just tell me if you have seen Charlie Wilson."

"Yeah. He was in here a couple of minutes ago. Said he was going down to look at the operating room schedule. Say, how about dinner tonight?"

"Can't do it Pete. I've got a tough case at 7 o'clock tomorrow morning, which will require me to get here at 6:15 to set up. Thanks anyway. I'd better hurry if I am going to catch Charlie."

She found Dr. Wilson leaning over the OR supervisor's desk looking at the week's surgical schedule.

Dr. Wilson was 55 years of age, a graduate of Harvard Medical School, and knew more about what went on at Riverside Hospital than almost anyone. For some reason, he was one of those curious creatures who found it delightful to know everything about everyone's business. He didn't always have the facts right, as he was a prod-and-press gossip, but at least he'd get her started in the right direction.

"Got a minute?" Dr. Wolfe inquired.

"Sure. What's up?"

"Keep this under your hat, but I've been assigned to do a little snooping into the sour cases of Dr. Harold Silver. Anything come to mind?"

"Let me think." Dr. Wilson was a general surgeon with good skills. "I never use him on any of my cases, but I've heard that in the past year, year and a half, he's fouled up a couple of cases of Dr. Brown and one with Dr. DeGaugh. I bet if you check with the operating room supervisor, she'll know the names of the cases. Say, what time is it?"

"Quarter to 12."

"Wow! I've got to get ready for surgery. See you later, Ursula. Say, how about dinner tonight?"

"Sorry, Charlie. I like my men a little younger. Besides, I just turned down the best-looking surgeon in town because I've got a tough case tomorrow, so how could I say yes to you? Give me a raincheck."

After talking with the operating room supervisor, Dr. Wolfe had the names of the three patients Dr. Wilson had mentioned. She checked the list Dr. Grant had given her and found it included all three. She then located the doctors, Herman Brown and Francis DeGaugh, who convinced her that Dr. Silver was not a competent anesthesiologist. To them, he was not capable of handling anything except the most routine cases. She didn't get the details of the cases, but she trusted their judgment.

She talked further with the operating room supervisor, and with members of her staff, and found that none of them liked to work cases on which Dr. Silver was the anesthesiologist. It seemed that something always went wrong and it always took twice as long as it should. She made a few notes and decided to talk to Anderson, the administrator, as soon as her 1 o'clock surgery was completed. She was looking forward to this case. It was open-heart surgery with Dr. Strong and Dr. Samuel Carver, two of the best cardiac men at Riverside Hospital. It was always a pleasure to work with good surgeons.

As the surgeons finished closing, Dr. Wolfe pulled off her surgical mask and congratulated them on a good case. She had performed her job well and no one could say that her work wasn't A-1 today. She looked at her watch: 4:30. Wow, was that a long case! She decided to catch a tuna salad in the cafeteria and then look for Anderson. Dr. Grant joined her.

As she sorted through her salad, she discussed the three cases with him. He asked if she had investigated Dr. Wilfred Harrison's two cases with Dr. Silver that were on his list. He told her what he knew about the cases and she made a few notes. Dr. Wolfe looked at her watch, then quickly excused herself. If she didn't catch Anderson before 5:30 he might be gone for the day. She grabbed her tray, put it on the conveyor belt, and hurried out toward the administrative wing.

Anderson was out of the office but was expected back at any time. Nonetheless, she asked his secretary to have him paged. Anderson did not answer the page. Dr. Wolfe waited a few minutes, then decided to catch him the next day. She wrote a note, centered it on his desk, and left.

Anderson had been attending a meeting of adminstrators of some of the area hospitals. The meeting was to have ended at 4:30 but did not finally wind down until 5:30. After the meeting ended, he began discussing problems in removing incompetent doctors from the medical staff with the administrators of Hilltop and People's hospitals. They did not identify any doctors by names.

The administrator of Hilltop Hospital told of an anesthesiologist who had been on the staff at his hospital whom everyone thought to be incompetent. It was not until several persons on the staff had written reports about one incident that the Credentials Committee had enough ammunition to initiate disciplinary action. It appeared that he had arrived for surgery under the influence of drugs. A nurse had found him unconscious. The surgery could not be postponed, and attempts to obtain another anesthesiologist were time consuming, delaying the operation almost four hours. The Credentials Committee finally had acted after that incident and the doctor did not fight to remain.

It was almost 7 o'clock when Anderson was ready to leave. He called his office for messages and went home to forget all about the hospital and Dr. Silver.

* * * * *

The next morning when Anderson arrived at work, he found Dr. Wolfe's note:

> Mr. Anderson,
>
> I think we have enough to hang Dr. Silver. I'll talk to you Friday afternoon about my findings.
>
> *(s) Dr. Wolfe*

He pushed the note aside and spent the rest of the morning running his hospital, not thinking of Dr. Silver. By afternoon he was winding up his work in preparation for his big weekend and by 3:30 was ready to depart. Dr. Silver's name had not crossed his mind all day, except when he saw the now-forgotten note.

Anderson knew it was after 3:00 because the sun now was shining in his office window. He was sitting behind his large mahogany desk, tidying it up and thinking about getting away early so he and his wife could start out. They had been invited up to the lake, several hours drive away, by an old college pal, Bud Davis, who had a place there. Anderson was looking forward to spending a relaxing weekend boating and fishing with the Davises. He and Davis had met their wives while all were students at the university and Martha and Anne were sorority sisters. The couples had married following graduation and had kept in close contact ever since. Davis was a reporter for a big-city daily and did occasional articles on the health care field.

Anderson admired his tidy desk and well-appointed office. He hated the cluttered look of many of his fellow administrators. He though cluttered desks indicated that executives didn't know what they were doing and didn't have a handle on the situation. He always wanted it to look as though he knew what was going on and was well on top of any situation. It was 3:35 and he decided to leave. He put on his coat and approached the door. It opened abruptly and in burst Dr. Wolfe.

"Fred, I'm glad I caught you. I finished my investigation and I wanted to get that off my mind so that I could enjoy the weekend."

Her last comment and the way she delivered it indicated to him that there was no way he could put her off until Monday. So he turned, motioned her to sit, and plopped down into his Moroccan leather chair.

"What did you learn?"

"Fred, I learned that Dr. Silver is a menace in the operating room. I've got five cases that he worked on in the last 18 months where he completely botched the whole affair."

"Have you got this in a written report, Ursula?"

"Oh, no, not yet. I haven't had time. But I'm not sure we need a written report." She pulled her notes from her white physician's coat and spread them out on Anderson's desk.

"Can I get you anything to drink, Ursula?"

"No, thanks, Fred. This won't take but a minute." Dr. Wolfe reviewed what she considered to be the three worst cases of those she had discovered and watched approvingly as Anderson seemed to be making copious notes. The administrator looked at his watch. It now was 4:45. Oh, how Dr. Wolfe could talk! He decided to cut her off as the lake was waiting and, besides, he trusted her to be sure of her facts.

"Well, Ursula, I think you have done a great job. Why don't you write up your report and we'll take it to the chief of staff on Monday."

"Hey, wait a minute, Fred. I think that this guy is such a menace that you ought to suspend him tonight. I checked the operating room schedule. He's got a case on for Monday morning that looks like it could be a pretty serious one, three or four hours under anesthesia."

Anderson could feel the sweat run down the back of his neck. No way was he going to suspend Dr. Silver tonight. The case she was talking about was one in which Dr. Ginsberg, chief cardiologist (and golfing friend), was operating and he had been months putting it together. Dr. Silver was only a backup anesthesiologist, helping Dr. Fred Keaton.

"No, Ursula, I don't think we should do that. Dr. Silver's staff appointment expires at the end of next month and I think that the way we ought to handle this is not to renew his appointment. I've got a feeling that if we did that, he'd back away from the situation since he has at least three other hospitals where he can practice."

"Damn it, Fred. Dr. Strong was right. You don't have any balls. If I were in your shoes with these facts, I'd be on the phone right now jerking that guy's privileges!"

Anderson was from the old school and hearing a woman talk like that didn't convince him that he was wrong; he turned her off halfway through her conversation. He was angry when he said:

"Look, Ursula, now you're getting into my job. I'll take responsibility for this. I appreciate your comments but I think this is something that can wait until Dr. Silver's appointment expires.

"Come on, it's late, let's get out of here. We've got a big weekend ahead of us. Besides, I think when you reflect on it, you'll see I'm right. You drop a summary suspension on Dr. Silver, he would immediately invoke the appeals procedure and we'd still be fighting him at this time next year. No, I think that I am right.

"We tell him that we aren't going to renew his appointment and he'll shrug his shoulders and say 'So what. I've got two or three other hospitals at which I can practice. I've been spread too thin anyway.' I know this guy. I know how to read personalities. I haven't been in this business for nearly 30 years and not learned something about doctors."

Dr. Wolfe was brash, and occasionally less than articulate, but she wasn't stupid. She could see she was fighting a losing battle and decided to suppress her urge to tear into this weak male, go home, and maybe jog up to the park to think about the situation. Besides, maybe that nice-looking architect would be up there putting in his ten miles. It might be fun spending the evening talking about structures and stress.

* * * * *

The weekend went well. Anderson caught a dozen or so fish, and Dr. Wolfe found architecture much more interesting that she had ever imagined. The weekend refreshed her and the thought of fighting Anderson now seemed silly. She arrived early Monday morning and wrote a report on the Silver matter for Anderson.

> TO: Fred Anderson, Administrator, Riverside Hospital
>
> FROM: Ursula Wolfe, Chief Anesthesiologist, Chairwoman, Ad Hoc Committee on the Investigation of Dr. Silver
>
> DATE: June 2, 1977
>
> The Schultz and Smith cases of Dr. DeGaugh and the Blue case of Dr. Brown were reviewed and discussed with Drs. DeGaugh and Brown. Also discussed these cases with operating room nurses. Based on this investigation, I find that Dr. Silver is not competent to handle other than routine cases. I would not recommend him for reappointment to the Riverside Hospital staff.

She looked at her signature and thought to herself, I need to get a new pen to have a bolder expression in my signature. She wondered how her signature would appear on Presidential stationery. She had thought how great it would be to be the first woman President of the United States. She would be 35 this year but she had been born in Germany. She conceded that another woman would have to suffice unless she could change the Constitution. That was a thought.

She grabbed her report and started toward Anderson's office.

Anderson walked into the hospital looking very relaxed. He had brought a couple of fish for the cook to serve at the Executive Committee meeting today. It was 7:30 A.M. and his secretary had not yet arrived. He took out his keys, opened his door, and admired his office. As he stepped in, his foot made contact with a piece of paper that had been slipped under the door. He bent down, picked it up, and noticed it had typing on it. He put on his glasses and saw it was a report from Dr. Wolfe. Not very long, he thought, but she's positive in her conclusion. He sat down behind his desk, got up again to get a cup of water for his African violet, then called the operator to see if she could locate Dr. Strong, the chief of staff. He started back through the mail he hadn't finished on Friday when Dr. Strong walked into his office.

"What's on your mind, Fred?"

Anderson handed the report to Dr. Strong and said, "The Ad Hoc Committee on the investigation of Dr. Silver has concluded that we ought to get him off the staff."

"It's all right by me, Fred. I'd never have that guy work on any of my cases. Do we need to have any meetings?"

"Sure, we'll have to refer this to the Credentials Committee and have it act on his reappointment with the other July candidates. I'll review the procedure and prepare the necessary paper work. I'll let you know what action is required on your part."

"Okay, Fred. I'd better finish my rounds. See you at lunch today."

Anderson pushed the button for his secretary. Maude collided with Dr. Strong as she responded. "Excuse me, Dr. Strong," Maude said, smiling, as their bodies made contact. Dr. Strong made a mental note to thank Fred later. Maude was blushing when she entered the office.

"Yes, sir?"

"Maude, get me a copy of the medical staff bylaws. I've got to figure out the technicalities of reappointment."

"Should I call Mr. Little?"

"Oh, that won't be necessary, Maude. Arnie Little charges 125 bucks an hour for legal advice and I think I'm smart enough to read the medical staff bylaws."

Maude returned with a current copy of the bylaws and put them on Anderson's desk. He had left to go down to the Medical Records Department to inspect the three cases Dr. Wolfe had mentioned in her report. When he arrived in Medical Records, he learned from Sara Kirts that Mrs. Helen Bellows, the head of the department, was ill. He asked Miss Kirts if she had been present when Dr. Wolfe had received some files last week. She said she had seen Dr. Wolfe come in but did not know what she had wanted. She was sure that Mrs. Bellows would know. The administrator decided against calling Mrs. Bellows at home and went back to his office to review the medical staff bylaws.

The bylaws indicated that the reappointment recommendations were the responsibility of the Credentials Committee. That panel's recommendations were made directly to the hospital's Board of Trustees at the monthly meeting prior to the expiration of the medical staff year. Recommendations concerning staff physicians were based on the information received from the chief of staff and the chief of the department to which the doctor was assigned. Any additional information the Credentials Committee deemed appropriate, including any statements by other members of the staff, could be considered.

Anderson reached for the phone and asked the operator to page Dr. Roger Connors, an orthopedic surgeon who took care of the football team at River Valley Community College. Most importantly, Dr. Connors was the chairman of the Credentials Committee. The phone rang. The operator reported that Dr. Connors did not answer the page, and asked if he should call his office. Anderson said that would be fine and to call him back. He then forgot about the call. Anderson never had problems erasing work from his mind when he left the office. The reverse was not true, however.

In his in-basket was the latest edition of "Fishing." He started thumbing through it. His thoughts flashed back to the past weekend and he revelled in the thought of the looks on faces of the Executive Committee members at noon when they learned they were eating fish freshly caught by the hospital administrator. The phone rang and the operator had Dr. Connors on the line.

"What's on your mind, Fred?" Dr. Connors blared. He was a giant of a man with a giant of a voice. Perhaps big voices and orthopedic surgery go together, as witness Dr. Bill Grant.

Anderson held the phone a couple of inches from his ear and said, "How are you coming on next month's reappointment list?"

"I don't know. We meet tomorrow afternoon."

"You guys better put your act together, we've got a problem with Dr. Silver. I've got a report here from the chief of anesthesiology recommending that he not be reappointed to the staff."

"What's our timing with the Board of Trustees?"

"Well, the board meets the third Thursday of every month, which is two weeks from this Thursday."

"Fred, make sure that I get a copy and I'll bring it up at the Credentials Committee tomorrow."

"Okay, I'll have a runner take it over to you in a few minutes."

"Thanks. See you later."

* * * * *

At the meeting the next day, Dr. Connors handed Drs. Bernard Arnold, Wilfred Harrison, Theodore Smith, and Charles Perkins copies of Dr. Wolfe's report and a list of the doctors whose medical staff years expired in July.

"Say, Roger," Dr. Arnold asked, "do we have anything on any of the doctors except Silver?"

"Not that I know of. Any of you other guys have any thoughts on the doctors on the list?"

"No, they look okay to me," Dr. Smith said. "I move we recommend all of the doctors on the list for reappointment with the exception of Dr. Silver, and that we assign him to Drs. Harrison and Perkins for investigation, to report at the next Credentials Committee meeting."

"I second," Dr. Harrison said.

"No deal," Dr. Connors cut in. "We've got a timing problem. Fred Anderson indicates that we can't let any grass grow under our feet on Dr. Silver and that we need prompt action."

"Well, for my money," Dr. Perkins said, "I've never seen a chick more sure of herself than Dr. Wolfe. I doubt if we are going to come up with anything more than what she's found.

"O.K.," Dr. Smith said, "I'll withdraw my motion."

"Fine," said Dr. Perkins. "Then I'll make a motion that we recommend reappointment for everyone except Dr. Silver and that we recommend that he not be reappointed."

"On what grounds?" Dr. Arnold asked.

"On the basis of Dr. Wolfe's report."

"I second the motion," Dr. Arnold said. It was passed unanimously.

"Okay, got anything else, Roger?"

"No, that's it," Dr. Connors concluded.

Dr. Connors picked up his notes and the information on Dr. Silver and walked into Medical Records.

"Say, Mrs. Bellows, can you have one of your gals type up the minutes of the Credentials Committee meeting we just concluded?"

"Sure, tell me what you want."

"Well, here is the list of doctors. We approved everyone but Dr. Silver and agreed to not recommend him for reappointment on the basis of Dr. Wolfe's report. Put a copy in my box and put the original of the minutes on Fred Anderson's desk. Thanks, Mrs. Bellows."

"You're welcome, Roger."

> Minutes of the Credentials Committee meeting of June 3, 1977:
>
> Chairman Connors called the meeting to order and stated that the purpose of the meeting was to review the doctors whose medical staff

years expired in July. Following discussion, upon motion of Dr. Perkins, which was seconded by Dr. Arnold, and unanimously carried, the Credentials Committee recommended that all doctors on the attached list be recommended for reappointment to the Riverside Hospital Medical Staff, with the exception of Dr. Harold Silver, since it was the recommendation of the committee that Dr. Silver not be recommended for reappointment on the basis of the report of the Chief of Anesthesiology, Dr. Ursula Wolfe, a copy of which is attached.

Respectfully submitted,

/s/*Roger Connors,* M.D.
Chairman, Credentials Committee

* * * * *

Dr. Strong and Anderson were sitting in the administrator's office having gin and tonics from the well-stocked bar built into the credenza behind the executive's desk. He had a small refrigerator and some expensive glasses. Oh, how he hated to drink out of those plastic throwaway glasses that the hospital used. He loved to hear the tinkle of ice as it struck the side of a good highball glass. He held his drink up and said,

"Salute, Bill! Thank God for the British! If it wasn't for a little gin, I don't know how we'd ever get through the summers here in the Mississippi Valley. Hell, if Kipling would have come here instead of India, Old Man River would have been in the King's English."

"What are you talking about?" Dr. Strong asked. "Tell me what I've got to say in my report to the board this Thursday."

"Just present the report of the Credentials Committee and indicate that Ursula Wolfe made a thorough investigation and that it is in the best interests of the hospital not to reappoint Dr. Silver."

"You don't think that I have to say anything more than that?"

"No. The board understands that it has to rely on the medical staff regarding the competency of its members."

"Well, here's to Kipling."

"Now, why did you say that, Les?"

"Hell, I don't know. You're the one who brought him up."

Anderson was right. The board didn't ask any questions and approved the report of the Credentials Committee and an implementing motion. The board directed Anderson to write to all of the doctors reappointed to the staff, notifying them of that action, and to notify Dr. Silver that he was not reappointed and to so advise the secretary of the medical staff of the board's action. Following is the letter Anderson wrote to Dr. Silver:

RIVERSIDE HOSPITAL
Office of the Administrator

June 20, 1977
Dr. Harold Silver
1929 Barge Street
Riverside

Dear Dr. Silver:

This is to advise you that the Board of Trustees of Riverside Hospital at its regular meeting held on June 19, 1977, did not reappoint you to the medical staff. Your appointment and privileges to admit and attend patients at Riverside Hospital will terminate as of August 1, 1977.

Yours very truly,

/s/Fred Anderson
Administrator

Anderson signed the letter and looked up to see Dr. Wolfe standing in the doorway.

"Well, Fred, do you think that we will get any static from Dr. Silver?"

"I don't think so, Ursula. He's on the staff of three other hospitals in town. He doesn't do enough work here to worry about."

"Well, I'm a little concerned because I just found out that he's lost his privileges at Hilltop and St. Francis. That leaves only People's where he has privileges."

"I didn't realize that," Anderson said. "Looks like we didn't act too soon. What seems to be the problem?"

"I don't know. The scuttlebutt is that Dr. Silver has a drug problem. Do you know anything about that?"

"I'm not aware of it," Anderson replied. "You're the one who supervises him. What do you know about it?"

"Well, I never thought the guy was with it, but I never suspected drugs. Maybe that explains the situation."

Anderson thought back to the conversation he had had with the Hilltop administrator. Maybe Dr. Silver was that anesthesiologist.

Dr. Wolfe suddenly said, "Well, anyway, I feel confident that we did the right thing. I've gotta run, I've got a soccer game to referee."

"I thought the schools played soccer in the spring. Hey, by the way, schools aren't in session now. What soccer game?"

"Oh, it's a men's semipro league. It gives me something to do, and besides, it upgrades the quality of the game. Those clowns don't know the rules and they need a little education once a week from me. See you later, Fred."

* * * * *

Several days later Maude hurried into Anderson's office and laid a letter from a Ronald Sampson on his desk, saying, "I think you may want to look at this, Mr. Anderson."

"In a minute, Maude, in a minute. What is it anyway?"

"It's a letter from a lawyer about Dr. Silver."

Anderson snapped around. What was going on? He didn't like the urgency in Maude's voice. He walked over to his desk and looked at the letter.

> June 23, 1977
> Dear Mr. Anderson:
>
> My client, Harold Silver, M.D., advised me that he was not reappointed to the medical staff. The letter he received set forth no reasons for the Board's failure to reappoint.
>
> We would like a statement of the reasons for the Board's action, so that we may initiate an appeal pursuant to Section 8 of the Medical Staff bylaws. Your prompt written response will be appreciated.
>
> Your very truly,
>
> */s/Ronald Sampson*
> cc: Harold Silver, M.D.

"Maude, get Arnold Little, our attorney, on the phone. I want to discuss this letter with him."

"Yes, Mr. Anderson, right away!" After a call she said, "He's not in."

"Hell, he's probably out playing golf. What time is it, Maude?"

"It's 2:30, Mr. Anderson."

"Thanks. Keep trying. Mr. Little has got to get this cleared up. I don't want this thing to ruin my weekend."

"Yes, sir, but it's only Tuesday."

"I know, Maude, but this doesn't look like an easy problem to me."

* * * * *

Little returned Anderson's call the next morning and was told about the letter.

"What's the doctor's name again?" Little said. "Silver? So, tell me again what happened."

Anderson did so.

"Okay, okay," Little said. "Before we write the letter to Ron Sampson let me come over and talk to Dr. Wolfe to see what should go in the letter."

Dr. Wolfe met with Little in the afternoon. Anderson, Dr. Strong and Dr. Grant also were present. Little started the discussion and soon pointed out that the investigation was skimpy at best and was lacking in specifics. He made his points forcefully. Dr. Wolfe interrupted: "Quit shouting, Mr. Little. I can hear you."

It was clear that she was resorting to the tactic she knew best: when in trouble, attack. She could see Little was right, that she had really not conducted an investigation. The attorney could discern that she had just put words in people's mouths and heard what she wanted to hear, rather than getting the facts and seeing whether she had witnessess willing to testify as to their knowledge.

Dr. Wolfe, when pressed by Little, conceded that Dr. Brown had said he wouldn't testify against Dr. Silver, although he had said that the anesthesiologist had botched his role in several of his cases. All of the nurses she had talked with had told her that they didn't want to be involved. What seemed to be such a good case against Dr. Silver wasn't so good when put to the test of an appeal.

"Well, what do you think we ought to do?" Anderson asked.

"What about the case that is pending against him and me?" Dr. Grant asked. "Hell, he really botched that one up."

"We can't go beyond Dr. Wolfe's report," Little said. "My suggestion is that I talk to Sampson and we see what he is driving at. He's always trying to strike a deal and maybe he's got something up his sleeve this time. Has anybody heard more about Dr. Silver?"

"I have," Dr. Wolfe said. "He's been bounced from the staffs of Hilltop and St. Francis. Somebody said he was using drugs."

"Any chance of his leaving town?" Little asked.

"I don't know. It's a possibility," Dr. Grant said. "I understand he has been to Oregon a couple of times in the last two months. Maybe he's looking for a new place to set up practice."

"Well, for our sake, let's hope that's what's happening," the attorney said. "I'm not sure we can make this failure to reappoint stick. I've gotta leave. I've got to be in court in 15 minutes. I'll get back to you, Fred, as soon as I can run Ron Sampson down."

The court to which Little referred was the racketball court. He had a regular Wednesday game with Don Thomas at 3:15 at the Riverside Athletic Club.

Later, Little was sitting in the steam bath nursing a cramped calf muscle that had cost him the match with Thomas. They played for $5 a game. He had won the first, then felt a little tired in the second and let Thomas win it. Then, trying to get a ball in the forecourt, he had fallen in pain when his calf muscle cramped. Not enough calcium, he suspected. He decided he'd switch to Kahlua and milk. It was too long to wait for the eggnog season. Well, as he chuckled about that, the door opened and much to his surprise in walked Ron Sampson. Hell, in the nude, Sampson didn't look like much. There was a true example of the clothes really making the man. Anyway, he thought he would make the most of the situation.

"Hey, Ron. What brings you in here?"

"Oh, I've taken up jogging, Arnie. I've got too much invested in my wardrobe to get that middle-age spread, and it seems to be the thing to do. Let me tell you, the best part of it is this steam. Sure helps the old aching muscles."

"You're telling me? My muscles cost me five bucks. I've got the worst cramp in my calf that I've had in 10 years."

"Not enough milk, Arnie. I take calcium pills. Stop by my locker before you leave and I'll give you some."

"No, thanks. I'm just going to switch to Kahlua and milk for my after-work pick-me-up."

"Say, Ron," Little said, changing the subject. "We got your letter over at Riverside Hospital and I'd like to know if you're really serious about going through with the appeal?"

"Sure we are. I don't think you had grounds to kick him off the staff. He may not be the best anesthesiologist in town, but as far as I know he's competent."

"Well, I wouldn't be so sure of that, Ron. We've got some pretty good evidence that says you're wrong. In fact, he's lost his privileges at a couple of other hospitals."

"I know that, Arnie, but we're appealing those, too. Somehow he's gotten a bad name and I think it's over the case he was just sued on. He's just a little different in personality and everybody was looking for an excuse to get rid of him. This town has got about the tightest clique of doctors I've ever seen anywhere. This group is getting so in-bred it will fall like the Roman Empire."

"Well, at least they're not eating off of pewter plates," Little said.

"Let me tell you, Arnie," Sampson said. "The truth of the matter is, Silver is going to leave town. He always wanted to do some sailing and Oregon really appeals to him. This riverboat stuff is not his cup of tea. He wants to unfurl the spinnaker and really get with it, if you know what I mean. I'll make you a proposition. Give us a promise that you'll reinstate him so we have a clean record for the Oregon hospitals, and we'll drop the appeal."

"No deal, Ron. But, I'll tell you what I will do. I'll get Anderson to agree that he won't give them the full nine yards when they ask for a recommendation."

"No, that's not acceptable. Wow! It's getting hot in here. See you later, Arnie. Let me think about it. I'll give you a call."

Little looked for the sponge and bay leaves and began working on his right calf again.

* * * * *

Little was in Anderson's office first thing Thursday morning and reported:

"Fred, here's the deal Sampson wants and it doesn't sound too bad. He says Silver is going to Oregon and all he's looking for is a chance to get on the staff of a hospital out in Portland. He says if we'll promise to sit on the Wolfe report and come up with some other reason for dropping him from the staff, he'll drop the appeal. Have you got any ideas?"

"Let's get Les Strong in here and see what he can think of. Besides, we'd better have the medical staff input in this deal. Maude, get the operator and have her page Dr. Strong. He's usually here. See if he can come down for a few minutes."

Dr. Strong saw Little in the administrator's office as he walked in and knew something was up. He listened intently as Little spoke, ending by saying, "That's the deal, Les. Have you got any ideas?"

"The only thing that I can think of is that when I was looking at the number of cases that Dr. Silver worked on in the last 12 months, I was surprised that he had only eight in all of 1976 and only four so far this year. Maybe we could say that we were trying to reduce our staff to those who really supported the hospital and he just didn't have enough cases, so we dropped him because he was interested in other hospitals and did most of his work elsewhere."

"Say, that's not bad," the attorney said. "What do you think, Fred?"

"That's really true. You know we are trying to get our staff to be more active and we are taking a hard look at those people who don't do much work here. We need to make some room for some of these interns and residents who are looking for a slot at our hospital when they finish training."

"Let's see if Sampson is in," Little said. "Let's use your speaker telephone in the board room, Fred."

The three went into the board room, where a picture of old Harvey Kutzer was staring down on them from the wall over the chairman's seat. Kutzer had been chairman of the board for 22 years, stepping down only last year. Anderson looked up at the old boy and smiled. Too bad he wasn't around. He would have had fun with this case. But, for some reason, it didn't seem fun to the administrator.

Little put in the call to Sampson. He was in and his receptionist put him on the line.

"Hello, Arnie, what's up? Get off that damn conference phone!"

"No, we are having a conference. I'm sitting here with Mr. Anderson, the administrator of Riverside Hospital, and Dr. Strong, the chief of staff. We want to see whether or not we've got a deal."

"Well, tell me what your proposition is."

"We'll agree that if you will withdraw the appeal, we'll state in response to any requests for information on Dr. Silver that he was not reappointed to the staff because it was the hospital's policy to limit its staff in the last two years to those who actively supported the hospital and Dr. Silver worked on only 12 cases in the last 18 months, which did not qualify him for reappointment."

"That doesn't sound too bad. Let me talk to Harold and I'll get back to you."

"Thanks, Ron. See you later. Bye."

"I think we've got a deal," Little said.

"Say, Arnie, what happens if Dr. Silver botches up a case in Oregon and the other hospital sues us for not shooting straight with them on his competency?" Dr. Strong asked.

"Hell, I've never read a case like that, Les. Don't worry about it. It will never happen." Anderson looked up at the picture of Kutzer.

* * * * *

(One year later.)

"I'm sorry, Mr. Little is out for the afternoon."

"What golf course is he on? I need to talk to him right away."

"I'm sorry, Mr. Anderson, I don't know. I'll let you speak with his secretary."

"Jane Thompson speaking."

"This is Fred Anderson at Riverside Hospital. I've got to get in touch with Mr. Little. Would you reach him and have him call me? No, it can't wait. I need to talk to him as soon as possible."

Shortly afterward, Little called back:

"Fred, what's wrong? Make it quick, I've got a couple of turkeys waiting for me on the 10th green. We're so far up they decided to press us at this point. Boy, my game's hot."

"Your game may be hot but I've got real troubles down here. I just got a notice to have my deposition taken by some Oregon attorneys who have a case against Dr. Silver."

"Hm, that doesn't sound good. Send the notice over to my office and I'll look at it tonight. I've got to go down there to get ready for a meeting in the morning."

Little decided to call the attorney in Oregon and see what he was up to with the deposition. He learned that the lawyer had been made aware of the suit the Chinns had brought against Dr. Grant, Dr. Silver, and Riverside Hospital and wanted the facts in that case to see whether he could turn up any witnesses on Dr. Silver's competency.

Little explained this to Anderson and instructed him that at the deposition he should tell them just what he knew about the Chinn case and let it go at that. There was nothing to worry about, he told the administrator.

* * * * *

It had been six months since Anderson had given his deposition. Everybody was gathered in the cafeteria for the annual Christmas party at Riverside Hospital. Anderson noticed Ursula Wolfe, Bill Grant, and Les Strong chatting by the eggnog with Arnie Little. Little was on his third cup of eggnog—he wanted to make sure he got enough calcium. He had a game with Thomas next Wednesday.

Dr. Grant looked over his scotch and water and noticed a man coming in the door. He didn't think he was a hospital employee but somehow he looked familiar. The stranger looked around and asked Mrs. Bellows a question. She nodded toward the punch bowl and the man started toward their group. Just as the man got to Anderson, Dr. Grant remembered when he'd seen him before: one and a half years ago at the golf course. He was a process server.

"Are you Mr. Fred Anderson?" the process server asked.

"Yes, I am."

"Here are some papers for you. Merry Christmas!"

OCEAN VIEW HOSPITAL OF PORTLAND, INC.,	)	
	)	
Plaintiff,	)	
	)	
v.	)	COMPLAINT
	)	
RIVERSIDE HOSPITAL AND FRED ANDERSON	)	
	)	
Defendants	)	
	)	

...FAILURE TO DISCLOSE PERTINENT INFORMATON REGARDING DR. HAROLD SILVER...

PRAYER IN THE AMOUNT OF $3,500,000.00

Commentary

THE STUDY

1.

Only after the filing of the Oregon lawsuit did Riverside Hospital realize the seriousness of its errors in handling the Silver case. There had been a lack of confidence in the medical staff bylaws and, as a consequence, an inability to effectuate their purposes. There also was a lack of appreciation for, and use of, candor by everyone involved. Dr. Silver had committed enough professional errors that any hospital, in any state, regardless of the adequacy of its medical staff bylaws, could have removed him from its staff. Riverside Hospital has a potential liability of $3.5 million because of its "careful handling" of Dr. Silver.

The facts allude to complicated medical staff bylaws. The truth was the opposite. The bylaws were workable. The hospital's failure was in not complying with them. The bylaws included the procedure for summary suspension. Anderson was properly reluctant to invoke that procedure based upon the scant facts he had at the time Dr. Wolfe made her oral report and requested summary suspension of Dr. Silver's privileges.

Anderson did not like the appeal provisions because he had been unsuccessful in the previous case. His failure to understand why he was unsuccessful resulted in his second-guessing Dr. Silver's attitude. Appeal procedures are bypassed only by physicians who, realizing the strength of the case against them, decide not to press the issue.

The appeal procedures were placed in the bylaws to ensure that, before taking action, the hospital gathered sufficient facts to justify resort to the disciplinary proceedings. Anderson apparently did not learn from the loss of the earlier case that the hospital must conduct an adequate investigation. Instead, he distrusted the process in the bylaws and attempted a shortcut.

The shortcut was in appointing the Ad Hoc Committee. Actually, there wasn't even a committee; Dr. Wolfe was off on her own investigating. Competent physicians are not always competent investigators. The hospital had no written policies on how to conduct investigations and gave Dr. Wolfe no guidance. When the hospital decided to check into sour cases, an audit should have been conducted. Like most good sets of bylaws, Riverside's provided for such an audit and for disciplinary action against doctors as a result of problems thus disclosed. Dr. Silver's errors, which Dr. Wolfe investigated, were of the type that would have been disclosed by an audit of his cases. The Ad Hoc Committee investigation should have been used only to supplement the audit. In this case, the Ad Hoc Committee procedure was a farce and only compounded other problems.

Dr. Grant's emotional appeal forced the administrator into a position of acting too quickly. Dr. Wolfe started her investigation with the idea of dumping Dr. Silver, rather than of getting facts. A good investigation must be comprehensive and impartial. Her investigation product was woefully inadequate. It definitely was not complete enough to support a negative recommendation, given Dr. Silver's potential for challenge. It is essential to do more than merely talk with people involved with a physician whose work is being scrutinized for possible disciplinary action or denial of reappointment. Once information comes to light through conversational channels, it is mandatory to obtain written statements that present with specificity the failings upon which the institution may base a negative determination.

Many persons are reluctant to reduce to writing what they are very willing to discuss orally. Only after their comments are in writing do they appreciate the need for complete accuracy. Writing necessarily involves a summary of the conversations that it confirms. Had Dr. Wolfe required signed statements, their content would have been available, and at a hearing oral testimony could bolster the case she had prepared. Witnesses have difficulty denying they have said something an investigator obtained in writing from them. Too often they will refuse to admit the substance of a conversation that had not been reduced to writing and signed by them. The writing commits witnesses to an unchangeable position.

The quality control procedures in the bylaws also were ignored. Once Dr. Wolfe made her initial report to the administrator, the next stage of the investigation should have begun, including a detailed review of patient charts.

The Credentials Committee, in the effort to save time, did not conduct its own independent investigation, as provided for in the bylaws. The report of the Ad Hoc Committee should have been the basis for a detailed, comprehensive investigation. Time is saved in disciplinary procedures when adequate investigations are conducted; time is wasted when action is taken on recommendations not well supported by evidence. An independent investigation by the Credentials Committee would have overcome the weaknesses of Dr. Wolfe's probing and could have brought out the facts needed to remove Dr. Silver.

The activities of the Credentials Commitee, if conducted properly, are another means of quality control. The committee's minutes did not contain the minimum information needed to support the recommendation. Dr. Wolfe's inadequate report could not be a proper basis for such action. When the minutes were presented to the board, they should have been accompanied by a complete report of the Credentials Committee, which had been approved by the chief of staff. Dr. Strong, chief of staff, like most of the others in the Silver case, felt uncomfortable becoming involved in the disciplinary process. The result was that the board, like the Credentials Committee, did not hear facts but rather accepted opinions based upon inadequate information.

Had the bylaws been followed, the hospital almost certainly would not have made the settlement that resulted in its being sued.

2.

Good communication techniques are rarely appreciated. The hospital's lawyer, Arnold Little, was in the business of preparing cases. He should have been notified and asked either to conduct or to direct the investigatory steps so that a useful record would be available. That record would have provided a documented basis for the board's negative determination on Dr. Silver.

The damage had been done before the hospital sought Little's counsel. After the letter was sent, there was hardly anything he could do. After his meeting with Dr. Wolfe and her sources of information, he determined that there was little basis in fact to justify the board's action. Had he been called in to supervise the investigation, or merely to review its results before the letter was sent, the outcome could well have been different. At that point he was looking to strike a deal to try to rid the hospital of Silver. The only other option would be to start all over to prepare a solid case against Silver.

The lesson Riverside Hospital learned from the filing of the $3.5 million suit was to prepare each situation by the book to determine whether it had a case and, if it did, to make certain it would stand the test of an appeal. This is fair to the physician and to the hospital, and much less expensive.

THE ISSUES

1.

References play a significant, if not a vital, role in the initial determinations of whether to grant an appointment to the medical staff as well as the scope of clinical privileges to be given. If references provided by the chief of a training program or representatives of a hospital where the physician previously was (or currently is) on the medical staff are not reliable, the institution at which an appointment is sought will have difficulty making an accurate appraisal of the applicant. Yet it is a well-recognized fact that there is considerable reluctance to be candid in supplying information about a physician whose professional performance has been below standard or who has engaged in disruptive conduct.

The most frequent explanation for such reluctance is concern that those who furnish candid, negative references are likely to be sued, and perhaps found liable, for defamation or conspiracy, with resultant costs of time and legal expense. Methods are available by which hospitals may protect those who provide references in good faith. Applicants can be reviewed to authorize release of information and to agree not to sue individuals providing information in the absence of malice or bad faith. Legislation has been enacted in many states to provide immunity for producing information under such circumstances. In short, the risks of suit and, particularly, of liability, need not be, and are not, as great as often is feared.

It also is necessary to consider the harm that may result when information is not furnished in a candid and forthright manner. As the case study indicates, under some circumstances a suit could be brought against the hospital as well as against the individuals who provide an inaccurate or incorrect reference on its behalf, although as yet there is no reported decision dealing with this precise question. For example, hospital A relies upon a positive, but untrue, reference furnished by hospital B with which the physician applicant previously was associated, and grants an appointment and privileges. The physician then engages in malpractice on one of the first patients the doctor cares for in hospital A. In such a case, it would be possible to assert that hospital B in providing the incorrect reference had breached a duty owed to hospital A, which had acted in part upon the reference, and to a patient who suffered harm at the hands of the physician.

If a candid reference had been furnished, the argument would go, it would have led to a denial of appointment to the physician and prevented harm to the patient. By responding to an inquiry or a solicitation of a reference, the hospital providing the information (in this case, B) accepts a duty to the institution requesting the information and its patients (hospital A), and must carry out this duty in a reasonable manner.

The case study suggests that the risk of a suit based on breach of that duty exists. Hospitals may want to consider whether the costs involved in such litigation, which could involve payment to a patient harmed by the physician as the result of malpractice, might far outweigh the expense of defending a suit brought by a doctor because of a poor reference when there was substantial information to support such a reference.

2.

When a physician is notified that adverse action is contemplated or has taken place concerning medical staff appointment or the scope of clinical privileges, and an attorney is involved on the doctor's behalf, the lawyer's first step usually is an attempt at negotiation, seeking a compromise. This is not, in itself, necessarily good or bad. The result of such negotiation can be an arrangement that serves the legitimate needs of the hospital, the physician, patients, and the public. However, the hospital and the medical staff have a public responsibility that they cannot overlook. Accomplishing the removal of a problem physician from a hospital, when it is known that this individual may well be a serious threat to the health or life of other patients in future contacts at other institutions, may not fulfill responsibilities to the public.

Too many physicians have been allowed to move from institution to institution and from state to state, with their poor records hidden from responsible institutions or public agencies, because of negotiated settlements of medical staff problems such as the one in the case study. The hospital that "cuts a deal" that results in passing misleading information on to another institution as to a physician's past performance should not ignore the implications of its actions.

If a file of such adverse information exists, it may legitimately be questioned whether the bargaining power of the physician seeking acceptable references is as great as the doctor's attorney may indicate during the negotiation process. For example, the hospital board, administrator, attorney, and key members of the medical staff negotiate, or must agree to, a settlement concerning a physician whose performance has been unsatisfactory. In doing so, they may wish to reflect on how they would feel if they or a member of their family were to be placed under the care of a physician who had won a negotiated settlement at another institution that, as part of the deal, had provided a misleading reference, which in turn led to an appointment and privileges for the doctor at their own institution.

3.

It would appear appropriate for a hospital at which some disciplinary or corrective action has been taken against a physician to notify other hospitals in the community where the doctor has privileges of its action so they can consider whether, and to what extent, they should take disciplinary or corrective action. Ordinarily, on forms for appointment and reappointment, physicians must indicate all hospitals where they have privileges. Thus, it is not difficult to know where notice should be directed when such action is taken. In the case study, the two hospitals in Riverside that had dropped Dr. Silver were remiss in not informing Riverside Hospital of their actions.

4.

A hospital might well provide in its medical staff bylaws that medical staff members are under an obligation to notify it of any disciplinary or corrective action against them at any other institution with which they are associated within a specific time, such as 10 days, after the action has been taken. The burden should be placed upon the physicians to make known their difficulties at other institutions rather than the hospital's having to rely upon notification from the one involved, or informal channels of communication within the medical community. If physicians do not fulfill the obligation to notify the hospital of adverse action elsewhere, that silence itself could provide the basis for revocation or suspension of their appointments when the penalty eventually becomes known.

Notification alone does not necessarily entail corrective or disciplinary action. It alerts the hospital that it is necessary to gather information regarding the conduct upon which the disciplinary action is based. A hospital should not have to await a report from a physician about disciplinary or corrective action on an annual or biennial reappointment form. That could lead to a long delay between the time the conduct occurred at another institution and the time the information became available, thus permitting a physician to continue in a course of malpractice. Such a time lag can raise risks that can and should be avoided.

Case 3

Going Bare Can Get You Thrown Out at Some Hospitals As Well As Some Beaches

PERSONAE

Phil Cox, attorney and member of board of Hohokam Community Hospital
Bill Crenshaw, member of hospital board
Harry Ellis, Hohokam Community Hospital administrator
Tex Landry, chairman of hospital board
Joseph McCurdy, Superior Court judge
Gordon Miller, hospital attorney
Dr. Charles Ryan, member of hospital medical staff
Dr. Joseph Sabina, general practitioner on hospital staff, protagonist
Martin Slaughter, Dr. Sabina's attorney
Mrs. Polly Weiler, member of hospital board

Sunshine Flats isn't much of a desert city—not an El Paso, Albuquerque, or Phoenix. Its water is pumped from deep wells, and the water table is dropping. But the beer that gushes from the tavern spigots is cold and there is money to spend when the cotton is harvested.

The few doctors practicing in the Sunshine Flats Valley are on the staff of Hohokam Community Hospital. They wine, dine, and golf at the Montazona Country Club with the town's lawyers, bankers, insurance brokers, cotton farmers, and merchants, some of whom serve on the hospital's Board of Trustees. Hohokam is the only hospital show in town and to the trustees, board service is a serious matter. Although they sometimes have their differences, by and large the doctors and the trustees get along well.

Dr. Joseph Sabina was no newcomer to the practice of medicine in Gila, a town a dozen miles south of Sunshine Flats. For more than 20 years he delivered babies, lanced boils, sewed up lacerations, and did all the rest that goes with a general practice in a rural community. He was an able physician but temperamentally he was more a crackling Dr. Kildare than a gentle Jean Hersholt. He had his opinions. He was not a shrinking violet in letting everyone know just where he stood.

Dr. Sabina's record at Hohokam Hospital was clean. His privileges had been renewed year after year without special restrictions. The peer review process had left him unscathed. He was regarded by some as a maverick whose strong suit wasn't gracious diplomacy but no one considered him a bungler.

He well knew that being competent and reasonably conscientious as a physician was no innoculation against malpractice lawsuits. He had been sued for claimed malpractice at least three times in recent years. A couple of these claims had resulted in compromise settlements, although they were of questionable merit. The insurance companies and their lawyers, he learned, dealt in probabilities and anxieties about jury sympathies, and possible boxcar verdicts, and not in resolute convictions about absolute rights and wrongs. His experiences with the judicial system and lawyers ranked the legal profession low in his esteem.

For years Dr. Sabina had carried professional liability insurance. Like auto insurance, it was something he had without a lot of thought. Then things began to happen with malpractice claims and insurance. The company that insured him stopped writing new policies. Then it went into receivership.

The other company that insured most of the doctors in the state had rejected Dr. Sabina's application for coverage and already had given notice of its intended withdrawal from the malpractice insurance market. A full-blown crisis had erupted. Not only had the cost of malpractice insurance skyrocketed but also it appeared that soon physicians wouldn't be able to get it even if they were willing to pay the price.

The state medical association did not accept the insurance crisis with philosophic resignation. After cursing the courts, the lawyers, the insurance companies, and many others, the association's organized effort for remedial action was a marvel to behold. Armed with reports of actuaries, lawyers, and insurance experts, its members converged on the legislature. After preparing the soil of public opinion with countless hours of explaining physicians' plight at service clubs, civic meetings, and to anyone who would listen, it was no surprise that the public opinion survey the group ordered resulted in a showing of broad support for its proposals.

The legislature came to the rescue. Malpractice tort reforms were instituted, including a claims screening panel. The state medical association was authorized to form its own malpractice insurance company with a state-backed joint underwriting plan providing low-cost excess coverage.

* * * * *

Meanwhile, by letter to Harry Ellis, the administrator of the hospital, Dr. Sabina gave notice that he was not renewing his malpractice insurance. It wasn't long before he had the administrator's reply: he would be suspended from the staff if he failed to conform to the medical staff bylaw requiring coverage of at least $250,000. The gauntlet was down and the stage was set for confrontation.

To Ellis, the matter was clearcut. The bylaws required insurance. If Dr. Sabina dropped his coverage, then he ought to be suspended, and that was that. Ellis's inclination to deal with problems directly and forcefully may have been a product of his frontier heritage but he accepted the recommendation of Hohokam's legal counsel that no suspension be imposed before the physician had an opportunity to be heard.

* * * * *

The hospital board scheduled a special meeting. Re-evaluation of the insurance requirement and the proposed suspension of Dr. Sabina upon the expiration of his policy were the key agenda items. Dr. Sabina was notified to attend the board meeting and he did, accompanied by his attorney, Martin Slaughter.

Tex Landry, the chairman of the hospital board, attempted to elicit from Dr. Sabina information about his assets and finances. Slaughter instructed his client not to answer, taking the position that a physician's financial status had no bearing on his qualifications to practice medicine in a hospital. Landry replied that Dr. Sabina's assets and finances had a bearing on whether he could afford liability insurance and whether he could contribute his fair share toward the payment of any judgment that might be awarded against both him and the hospital. The lawyer wouldn't budge from his position so the attempted probe into Dr. Sabina's finances never got off the ground.

Landry, as the area's leading Ford dealer, was accustomed to maintaining a pleasant smile. Although he appeared to accept with good humor the refusal of Dr. Sabina's lawyer to allow answers to his questions, the hardening of the lines at the corners of his mouth and eyes gave away the fact that he was genuinely annoyed, to say the least. His neck and face colored to a dark crimson, like the rising column of a thermometer, when the attorney asserted that the hospital board did not have the power to suspend Dr. Sabina because the staff bylaw provision requiring insurance spelled out no penalty for noncompliance.

"Cow pies," Landry blurted. "You are trying to walk us through cow pies," he said, shaking his finger at Dr. Sabina's lawyer.

Mrs. Polly Weiler, a board member, spoke up in an effort to calm the situation:

"We are straying off the point. We ought to be talking about whether we should stay with the insurance requirement, the pros and cons of it."

Landry was not diverted from his chagrin.

"I'll be damned if some pettifogging lawyer is going to tell me what we can't do to protect Hohokam," he declared. "What does he know about running this hospital, about staying within its budget? Everybody knows you don't run a business without insurance unless you're a fool. The hospital has insurance and the bylaws say the doctors are supposed to have it. Where does he come off telling us some doctor can break the rule and we can't do anything about it?"

Phil Cox was the only lawyer on the hospital board. He had practiced law in the valley for more than 25 years. He also held in partnership with his brother several sections in cotton and milo maize. For a lawyer he tended to be unusually quiet. It was his custom to listen and say little. When he spoke, he used few words, but people paid attention.

"We ought to let Doc have his say," he said.

Landry, somewhat embarrassed at having lost his cool, hurriedly agreed. He asked Dr. Sabina if he had anything he wanted to say to the board.

"Indeed I do," he replied. Without ceremony he launched into an explanation of his position.

He declared that a substantial number of his patients were unskilled stoop laborers with marginal earning ability. Many of these families, he contended, were able to maintain themselves at no more than a bare subsistence level, sometimes by keeping their children home from school to help with the picking of onions, carrots, melons, and lettuce. These people, he asserted, were not being provided with free health care because the county used an unrealistic means test for eligibility. These people, he went on, weren't able to pay for the health care they needed and it would make the situation worse to raise his fees to cover the escalating malpractice insurance costs.

Dr. Sabina's second major contention was that malpractice insurance was largely responsible for the proliferation of claims against doctors. The lawyers, he charged, were far more interested in dipping into deep pockets than they were in improving the practice of medicine. He cited an article he had read in support of the contention that doctors with no insurance were less likely to be the targets of malpractice lawsuits than those with large policies.

Bill Crenshaw, the local bank manager, was the newest member of the hospital board. He was less than eager to inject himself into the controversy, particularly since the hospital and several members of the medical staff were bank customers. Nevertheless, he commented that there was no way the hospital could operate without insurance to protect its assets. He noted that the assets were held in trust for the public and that if physicians on the staff dropped their insurance, it would be more likely that the hospital would be sued when a patient was hurt by a doctor.

Mrs. Weiler chimed in that she felt the insurance requirement might not be such a good idea if it would limit the access of Dr. Sabina's patients to medical care. She had been a nurse many years ago, before she married Tom Weiler. She never quite developed the same warm feeling about the Weiler family's cotton acreage as she had for the nursing profession. At home on the Weiler ranch, she maintained a makeshift dispensary where she ministered to the hurts and illnesses of the farm laborers. It gave her great satisfaction when they referred to her in Spanish as the "doctor lady."

Cox diplomatically commented that he shared her concern about inadequate health care for the disadvantaged. But he resorted to his lawyerlike ways in adding that there was no evidence indicating that Dr. Sabina's carrying or not carrying malpractice insurance would have a material effect on the availability of health care in the area.

Landry joined with Cox in dismissing the physician's argument based upon financial concern about the poor but he did so less diplomatically. He insisted, as he put it, on calling a spade a spade. Nothing they did, he argued, was going to change the fact that the poor always had less of everything except, he added, children. But no one laughed at his attempt at humor.

He continued in a serious vein, saying that the hospital was there to serve the entire community and that its financial viability would be placed in jeopardy because one stubborn doctor decided to buck the insurance requirement. He added that Ellis, the administrator, had informed him that a major insurance company that insured hospitals in California had imposed a 20 percent rate increase on health care institutions that had no doctor insurance requirement.

Landry said that although the insurance companies may deny it, it stands to reason that if the hospital's insurance company is going to pay out dollars on claims that used to be paid by the doctor's carrier, then the institution's insurance costs are going to increase.

Cox, the attorney member, cemented the board's support for the insurance requirement by reporting a story he had heard about how a New Orleans hospital had been intimidated by what he called a "sweetheart deal" into agreeing to a huge damage settlement. Cox described the case:

An uninsured doctor on the hospital's staff had applied a cast too tightly to a patient's broken leg. The swelling against the cast cut off circulation to the leg with the result that it became gangrenous and had to be amputated below the knee. When the patient's attorney learned that the physician had no insurance, he offered a sweetheart deal that the doctor accepted in order to save everything he had worked for years to accumulate.

The doctor paid $25,000, which he raised from his savings and a loan against the cash values of his life insurance. The deal involved an agreement that for every dollar in excess of $200,000 the patient recovered from the hospital, the patient would return 50 cents to the doctor. The deal meant that if $250,000 or more was recovered from the hospital, then the physician would get all of his money back and the entire loss would be thrown on the hospital. As a result, the doctor became an ally of the patient's lawyer in blaming the hospital and its nursing staff for the development of the gangrene, and the hospital's insurance company paid more than $300,000 to settle the case.

It was clear following Cox's account that the board members who had not expressed themselves favored retaining the insurance requirement. Mrs. Weiler still had concerns about the effect of the high cost of insurance on the poor but said she would go along with keeping the requirement because she thought the doctors ought to be able to compensate their patients for legitimate injury claims.

The vote to retain the insurance requirement was unanimous.

* * * * *

When the hospital board confirmed that he would indeed be suspended when his insurance was dropped, Dr. Sabina filed suit. He asked the court to enjoin the hospital, its board, and the administrator from terminating his staff privileges because of lack of insurance. He also asked for an award of damages against the hospital and its administrator, Ellis.

In his court complaint Dr. Sabina alleged:

1. That a letter from the hospital administrator advised that his staff privileges would be suspended when his malpractice insurance coverage expired.
2. That his present insurance carrier had its operation restricted by the state and renewal of that policy would not give him any real protection.
3. That he had been rejected by the only other malpractice insurance carrier writing such insurance within the state.
4. That there was no contractual or liability reason for requiring him to carry malpractice insurance coverage and any bylaw requirement to that effect was arbitrary and capricious.
5. That although the administrator told him that insurance for staff members was required to avoid an increase in the hospital's own insurance rates, he had a letter from the institution's insurance company confirming that it did not require staff members to carry malpractice insurance.
6. That termination of his staff privileges would unreasonably interfere with his practice of medicine, would cause him to lose income, and would jeopardize the health of his patients.

7. That the announced suspension was unjustified and resulted from a malicious scheme on the part of the administrator to promote practice by specialists at the hospital by taking patients away from general practitioners.

In response, the defendants filed a motion to dismiss. The motion relied upon a federal district court case that upheld a hospital's right to require malpractice insurance. On the damages question, it relied upon a state statute that stated:

> A person who, in connection with a hospital's duties or functions, without malice and in good faith makes a decision or recommendation as a member, agent or employee of a hospital's medical or administrative staff or of one of its review committees, is not subject to liability for civil damages or legal action in consequence thereof, nor shall a hospital, its administrators or its directors be liable for such activities of any such person.

* * * * *

The case came on for an early hearing before Superior Court Judge Joseph McCurdy. Injunction cases are given priority over others so Dr. Sabina had his day in court without the usual tangle of delays.

As his first witness, Dr. Sabina's lawyer, Slaughter, called his client. Dr. Sabina's testimony supported many of the contentions in his complaint:

He was a licensed medical doctor in good standing. He had been on the staff of Hohokam Community Hospital continuously for more than 20 years. Several of his patients were in various stages of pregnancy. The loss of his privileges would jeopardize their health and welfare.

"If I am not allowed staff privileges," he asserted, "it will require my sending them to a hospital out of the community." He also maintained that since he was an independent physician, not paid by the hospital, the institution could not suffer any loss or liability by his sole acts. And he said he had not been sued for malpractice.

His testimony that he had never been the target of a malpractice claim was clarified on cross-examination. He admitted that several claims against him had been settled by his insurance carrier and that others still were pending against him, but he pointed out that none of these cases involved the hospital. He also admitted that malpractice insurance was available to him under the new state medical association plan, but he declared that he had no intention of applying for coverage because the rates were too high.

Over objections, he was allowed to testify to his opinion that the defendant administrator, Ellis, had acted maliciously and in bad faith in proposing suspension of his privileges because there was no emergency and the medical staff bylaws allowed such suspensions only in emergencies.

Dr. Sabina was followed to the witness stand by Dr. Charles Ryan, who had been on the Hohokam Community Hospital staff for 11 years. He testified that he had observed a pattern developing over the years in which Ellis attempted, through his position as hospital administrator, to remove some physicians from the staff without apparent justification. It was his belief that Ellis was trying to attract medical specialists to the area and to promote the success of their practices by restricting the privileges of the general practitioners or eliminating them from the staff altogether.

However, he admitted under cross-examination that he had no personal knowledge of Ellis's feelings toward Dr. Sabina. Although he felt the actions were wrong, he acknowledged that he knew of no personal malice by Ellis or any board member toward Dr. Sabina.

Additional questions to Dr. Ryan elicited the information that he had been called on the carpet for inadequate records and for poor preoperative and postoperative patient care. He also acknowledged that his being called to account by Ellis wasn't all harassment. He admitted that one of his reviewed cases involved a clear error, "a tragic error" as he put it.

When he declared that he considered Dr. Sabina to be a friend, Gordon Miller, the hospital's attorney retorted wryly, "You indeed are a good friend."

Slaughter, Dr. Sabina's attorney, sprang to his feet and shouted an objection to that comment. A reprimand from Judge McCurdy was followed by a short recess.

The mayor of Gila, a member of the Gila Town Council, and a patient also testified for Dr. Sabina. They said he was the only medical doctor in town and agreed that most of his patients were low-income farm workers. An increase in his fees resulting from increased malpractice insurance costs, they claimed, would be harmful to the health and welfare of his patients. They also confirmed that Hohokam Community Hospital was the only institution in the area that could serve the needs of his patients.

The witnesses for the hospital established that Hohokam was a private, rather than a government, institution. Board members testified to the factors they had considered in deciding to keep the insurance requirement. Admitted in evidence was a certified copy of the resolution adopted by the board after the meeting with Dr. Sabina and his attorney. It read:

> Resolved: that the insurance to be maintained by members of the medical staff in order to meet the membership requirements of the bylaws shall continue to be professional liability insurance with minimum limits of $250,000.00.

Ellis had never seemed lacking in self-assurance as the hospital's chief administrative officer. He was different when on the witness stand. He looked uncomfortable and it was obvious that he wished he were elsewhere. He said Dr. Sabina was eligible for continuing coverage with the insurance program sponsored by the state medical association.

Objections by Dr. Sabina's attorney to Ellis's testimony on the availability of insurance were overruled by the court. Slaughter's objections focused on the fact that the state malpractice insurance program offered only "claims made," not "occurrence," policies, which are superior and provide protection to the insured for an incident regardless of when the claim is made, even many years later. He contended that "claims made" policies were not proper insurance becausc of the usual time lag between when an "incident" occurred and a claim actually was asserted.

Ellis acknowledged that as administrator of the hospital he initiated the decision that Dr. Sabina should be suspended if he insisted on disregarding the insurance requirement. He denied having improper motives: "I don't harbor any malice or ill will toward Dr. Sabina."

Slaughter began his cross-examination of Ellis by handing him a letter from the hospital's insurance company. In the letter the underwriting manager for the carrier confirmed his telephone advice to Dr. Sabina that the company "does not care whether or not doctors in an insured hospital carry malpractice insurance." The manager wrote that he knew of no insurance company that required staff doctors practicing in a hospital to carry malpractice insurance as a condition to providing such protection for the institution.

Ellis acknowledged that a copy of this letter had been directed to him. He maintained, however, that the insurance agency had let him know, in no uncertain terms, that if the doctors on the staff dropped their coverage the cost of Hohokam's coverage would go up.

The administrator admitted that he had urged medical staff committees at the hospital to cut back on some of the surgical privileges that had been granted for years to old-timers on the staff and that he had caused at least two of them to resign. It was no secret that he favored stricter delineation of privileges, with increased emphasis on graduate medical education as the basis for granting access. It was not, he insisted, that he favored the economic success of specialists; it was simply a matter of improving patient care at the hospital. The doctors who were pressured into resigning from the staff, he said, should have left long before they did—one was too old to handle the responsibility of caring for acutely ill or injured patients and the other was chronically impaired by alcohol.

* * * * *

When both sides finished with their witnesses the court called for their arguments. Dr. Sabina's lawyer fired a barrage of challenges to the validity of the insurance requirement:

- The bylaws provision requiring malpractice insurance was unreasonable and arbitrary because the financial condition of Dr. Sabina's carrier was suspect and another carrier had rejected his application.
- It would be cheaper as a matter of economics for the hospital to include the medical staff under its coverage than to require the physicians to carry their own insurance.
- The American Medical Association House of Delegates had declared that physicians should be encouraged by local medical societies to carry adequate professional liability insurance but that such self-protection should not result from coercion by a hospital.
- A resolution recently adopted by the AMA urged that medical staff privileges should be limited or denied only for reasons of professional competence or ethical judgment.
- The Accreditation Manual for Hospitals of the Joint Commission on Accreditation of Hospitals stated that privileges were not to be denied on the basis of sex, race, creed, or national origin, or "on the basis of any other criteria lacking professional justification."
- Federal Medicare regulations governing hospitals required staff privileges to be extended to licensed physicians unless it was determined that they were not professionally competent or lacked ethical worthiness.
- The staff bylaws spelled out no penalty for a doctor's failure to comply with the insurance requirement and allowed cancellation or reduction of privileges only "for any valid disciplinary reason."
- The insurance requirement, in effect, was a financial means test for medical staff membership that offended public policy because it could deny physicians the right to practice their profession and deny the public medical care.
- The low income of the community served by Dr. Sabina meant that his patients would be unable to afford the increased fees necessitated by his higher malpractice premiums.
- The actions of the hospital were subject to judicial scrutiny because public funds were involved in its construction and because, as the only hospital in the area, it could drastically affect a doctor's economic well-being.

Miller, the hospital's attorney, in response conceded that the institution's actions might be subject to the court's review but he insisted that the scope of such a review was limited. A hospital board, he argued, is entitled to require liability insurance of physicians as a proper exercise of business judgment. After all, he said, it is not at all uncommon in the exercise of a responsible business judgment for property owners to require users of their property to carry suitable insurance. He cited building leases, construction contracts, and auto leases as examples. The requirement, he pointed out, did not ordinarily emanate from a determination that a particular tenant, contractor, or driver was incompetent; rather, it arose from the recognition that even the most competent can make mistakes that can result in catastrophic liabilities.

He turned then to arguing that the liability of hospitals arising out of their use by medical staff members was a legal and economic reality. Some of the largest malpractice settlements involved joint contributions by physicians as well as the hospital, he said. He cited a report by the National Association of Insurance Commissioners that stated that hospital-based incidents accounted for 80 percent of medical malpractice claims. He pointed to several court decisions holding that hospitals could be held liable for inadequate supervision of the competence of staff doctors even though such inadequacies often actually resulted from the fact that physicians on the staff did not carry out their peer review responsibilities.

Requirements that physicians who wished to use a hospital be competent and carry liability insurance were not inconsistent or mutually exclusive, Miller said. The governing board of the hospital, he went on, had the ultimate power and discretion to determine the granting and denial of privileges, and its management authority was absolute so long as it acted within the law. The courts, he said, should not interfere with the board's exercise of discretion unless its action was so unreasonable as to demonstrate a clear abuse of discretion.

Furthermore, the attorney said, the insurance requirement would not deprive the public of needed medical services. Surveys by the state's hospital association had established that most institutions had an insurance requirement and most doctors carried such insurance.

Hospital counsel asserted that the economic realities were such that if doctors went bare (lacked any insurance), the claimants would strive to make their cases against the insured hospital. The results, he declared, would be nothing less than disastrous. The uninsured doctor, as a joint defendant, would not be able to participate fairly in settlements. An article in *Medical Economics* had reported a 20 percent increase in insurance rates for hospitals that could not show that all their medical staff members had malpractice insurance.

Switching his fire to the damages claim, Miller maintained that the hospital board had acted within its permissible range of discretion in retaining the insurance requirement. If the requirement was valid, he argued, then the board clearly had the right to exclude Dr. Sabina from the hospital for violating its mandate. Dr. Sabina's position that the board was powerless to enforce the insurance requirement because no penalty for violation was spelled out in the bylaws was patently absurd, the attorney said.

He declared that the position of the board as the ultimate governing authority was the same for hospitals as for other corporations: boards had the right to set policies and to make reasonable rules. They were not obligated, he argued, to adopt a code of criminal justice spelling out specific penalties for the violation of each policy or rule.

Miller charged that the claim for damages was frivolous because it was based on the hospital's retention of the insurance requirement—which it had a right to do. Even if it was decided that the insurance rule was unlawful, he asserted, it was evident that Dr. Sabina had proved no damages because he had sustained none. It was true that he would be obliged to obtain malpractice insurance from the state medical association program, but it nevertheless was a fact that he still had coverage and that his practice at the hospital had not been terminated.

Finally, Miller stressed the peer review immunity statute. Its purpose, he said, was to encourage all involved in the review of hospital medical staff members to participate in the process without fear of reprisal so long as they acted in good faith. If the physicians, board members, or administrative personnel who participated in the monitoring of the medical staff could be saddled with liability for damages, or even the cost of defending lawsuits, then the whole process would be seriously impaired, he declared. Although Ellis, the administrator, and a few board members may have been irritated by Dr. Sabina's intransigence, there simply was no evidence of personal malice toward him or any motivation on their part other than a legitimate concern for the best interests of the hospital and its patients, the hospital's attorney concluded.

* * * * *

The evidence was in and the arguments were over. Attention focused on Judge McCurdy, who was prepared to issue his decision.

At this point, it was undisputed that there were then only two reported cases in the law books dealing with a hospital's insurance requirement. One case held that a government hospital could not require insurance as a condition for granting staff privileges because the law spelled out the requirements for staff membership and insurance was not one of them. The other case was a federal district court decision that concluded that:

> Requiring its staff physicians to carry insurance and to submit proof to the hospital of that fact is surely a reasonable exercise of financial responsibility on the part of the hospital.

In this instance, neither of the two earlier cases carried the day. The government hospital case did not apply because Hohokam was a private institution and its staff membership requirements were set by its board, rather than by statutes. The federal court case also did not quite make it because it was only a decision by a trial court, not by a court of last resort. So Judge McCurdy had to grapple with the problem on his own, free from controlling precedent.

He dealt first with the question of whether the court had jurisdiction—any right at all to review the decision of the governing board of a private hospital. He made short shrift of that one. It was after all undisputed that Hohokam was the only hospital in the Sunshine Flats Valley. A local doctor either was on the staff of Hohokam or he just didn't use a hospital. The state supreme court a few years earlier had ruled that the medical society's exclusion of a doctor was subject to review when it was shown that the association had monopoly control over the keys to the local hospitals—an "understanding" a physician couldn't get on an institution's staff unless he belonged to the society.

Since Hohokam admittedly was the only hospital that Dr. Sabina could use, the court didn't have much trouble in following the monopoly rule and in holding that the board's actions were subject to review. In any event, he reasoned, the threatened suspension was subject to review because it was contended that the hospital would not be following its own medical staff bylaws in imposing the suspension.

He reiterated that he was aware that Hohokam was a private, nonprofit hospital, built entirely from private funds, and that he was mindful of the general rule that the exclusion of a physician from staff privileges at a private hospital was not subject to judicial review. But this general rule, he said, did not apply where, as here, the hospital was the only one in the area available to the doctor and his patients, or where it was contended that the institution's bylaws were being violated.

Whether or not the insurance requirement was lawful presented a tougher question. Judge McCurdy recognized the conflicting interests involved. On the one hand the board was responsible for the preservation of the fiscal integrity of the hospital. On the other hand Dr. Sabina was the only general practitioner in his town. His patients were mainly people with low incomes.

The court recognized that the hospital's right to self-preservation was a matter of legitimate concern. But Judge McCurdy's comments indicated he had difficulty accepting the reality of predatory lawsuits, of claimants' lawyers zeroing in on defendants who had deep pockets rather than on those without insurance whose responsibility for the patient's injury was clear. He concluded, however, that the court's review must be narrow.

He ruled that Dr. Sabina had been accorded his procedural due process on the insurance requirement, but had been unable to persuade the hospital board that, because of his special circumstances, he should be exempted from the requirement. The requirement, Judge McCurdy said, was not arbitrary or capricious as a matter of law. He said the court could not ignore the realities: if a patient is injured in the hospital, the institution almost always will be joined as a co-defendant, regardless of who is at fault. The hospital, he held, has the right to take reasonable measures to protect itself and the patients it serves.

Judge McCurdy then turned to the damages claim. He noted that Dr. Sabina was correct in stating that the hospital's medical staff bylaws authorized the chief of staff or administrator to impose temporary suspensions only in cases of emergency. But, he said, the bylaws provisions relating to summary suspensions were in no sense a limitation on the power of the governing board to establish policies for the hospital and to enforce such policies. The board has broad discretion in exercising its authority over the granting and withholding of medical staff privileges, he declared, and the courts should not substitute its judgment for that of the board so long as it appears that a physician has been accorded basic procedural fairness and there is some rational justification for the board's action.

He was not unmindful, he said, that his ruling on the insurance requirement rendered moot most any claim by Dr. Sabina for damages. Nevertheless, he felt that it was in order to comment upon the state's public policy as evidenced by the peer review immunity statute.

He stated his view that the showing of malice or bad faith required to defeat immunity had to be interpreted in such a way as to encourage, not discourage, review of medical staff activities within the hospital. Such reviews, he said, involved time-consuming, unpaid work that was likely to generate bad feelings. He expressed concern that if unhappy reviewees could easily file lawsuits following adverse decisions, then peer review could become an empty formality, if undertaken at all. He therefore concluded that it was the legislature's intent to ban such lawsuits except where there was real evidence of actual malice.

He observed that a hospital was a place fraught with constant pressure and emergency, with anger, irritation, jealousy, and personal animosity to be expected in such an atmosphere, especially when peer review was involved. Malice and bad faith, he said, meant in this context a primary purpose other than safeguarding the hospital and its patients.

Judge McCurdy concluded by ordering the case dismissed. He declared that a great deal more evidence than that presented by Dr. Sabina would be required to overcome the purpose of the statute: to encourage good faith physician review without fear of reprisal by lawsuit. The clerk entered the judgment and with a rap of the gavel the court stood adjourned.

* * * * *

The lawsuit was over but the insurance question was neither gone nor forgotten. A few of the hospitals in the state's larger cities had backed off from an absolute insurance requirement. Some others modified their strict requirement because of apprehension that some of their doctors might shift their practices to the hospitals with no requirement or with a flexible standard. Word of the changes at some hospitals filtered down to staff members at Hohokam and it wasn't long before the whole subject started cropping up again at board meetings.

New information indicated that even when hospitals had no insurance requirement at all, the overwhelming majority of their physicians carried protection anyway so that the effect on the hospitals' loss experience was less than had been feared originally. However, the options on how to go about backing off from an absolute insurance rule seemed endless and each one appeared to involve opening up a new can of worms.

First of all, board members who were close to some of the physicians on a social basis reported that the doctors' views about the insurance rule were far from uniform. Some doctors who were believed to oppose the insurance requirement turned out not really to be opposed at all. They opposed the requirement's inclusion in the medical staff bylaws because they felt that recommendations for staff privileges should be based entirely on considerations of demonstrated competence and ethical worthiness. They did not oppose the board's maintaining an insurance rule by resolution or in the corporate bylaws. In fact, some felt that they did not wish to associate on cases with uninsured physicians and that, if any staff members were going to be allowed to use the hospital without insurance, such doctors should be identified to the rest of the staff.

The discussions at board meetings ranged from whether the insurance rule should be abandoned altogether, should be retained without exception, or should be subject to exceptions upon a showing of good cause to the board. If exceptions were to be allowed, then there were questions as to what, if any, alternate financial responsibility requirements should be imposed.

- Should uninsured doctors be required to show that they had the ability to compensate patients for just claims and to pay their pro rata share of judgments rendered jointly against them and the hospital, or against them and other doctors on the staff?
- Should they have to sign agreements pledging that they would pay their pro rata share of joint judgments?
- Should they have to sign agreements guaranteeing that they would not enter into sweetheart settlements whereby they would benefit from damages awarded against the hospital or other physicians on the staff?

- Shouldn't antisweetheart agreements be signed by the hospital and insured doctors as well as by the uninsured ones?

The questions are seemingly endless. The trial has long since ended. Dr. Sabina has been thinking longingly about retirement. Harry Ellis has moved on to a better position at a larger hospital. But at the Hohokam Community Hospital board meetings, the discussions about the insurance requirement have continued.

Commentary

1.

Hospitals have become more than places where physicians treat their patients. They have become agencies for airing the demands and expectations of health care consumers and providers, and the primary tribunals for the resolution of conflicts among those involved in the health care scene. The stakes in these conflicts often are high. Questions involving life and death, professional reputations, and big dollars are the order of the day. Issues such as who gets to do what—or who gets to use the hospital at all—are regular items on the menu.

Patient expectations, as perceived by the courts, are reflected in the mounting number of decisions holding that hospitals are accountable for the competency and qualifications of the doctors they accept to practice. A physician's license may be unrestricted so that it covers the whole spectrum of medical practice and its specialties. But the hospital that allows a doctor to practice anesthesiology, neurosurgery, or any other area of medicine or surgery simply because the individual has a license does so at its peril.

The courts are espousing the view that allowing a physician to use the hospital for neurosurgical practice or some other area of practice involving special risks and requiring special knowledge may constitute a finding by the institution that the doctor is qualified to carry out such practice. They are saying that the hospitals, through medical staff committees, have a legal duty to monitor and supervise the competence of staff members. For breach of this duty, both the hospital and the doctor who is accused of screwing up can be the targets of a judgment for big dollars in favor of a patient.

So it's not just the Joint Commission on Accreditation of Hospitals that is nudging hospitals to take a closer look at peer review practices. It also is joint judgments that are precipitating such scrutiny. It is this same specter of joint judgments that is causing some hospitals to take a closer look at insurance requirements for medical staff members.

2.

In an environment where malpractice insurance is available, albeit expensive, several court decisions have upheld the right of hospital governing boards to impose an insurance requirement. Some of the rulings have gone so far as to uphold legislatively imposed insurance requirements so that physicians who elect to go bare will be faced with losing their tickets to practice. The courts are saying that the hospital has the right to take reasonable measures to protect itself and its patients.

In the case study, Judge McCurdy had to face some of the ugly realities of the court system allowing reparations for injuries caused by another's alleged negligence. If a patient is injured while in a hospital, the institution's joinder in the case becomes more probable when the physician does not carry malpractice insurance, even when the finger of negligence appears to point directly and solely to the doctor.

In like fashion, the erring doctor's colleagues, such as the anesthesiologist, the surgical assistant, and the consultants, are apt to be included in the lawsuit when the physician goes bare. Damage claims are supposed to follow the individuals at fault but they sometimes also pursue the deep pockets as if drawn by a divining rod. Hospitals can't hide their assets in a trust or pack up for a sojourn in Tahiti, and so it is that their governing boards take a hard look before backing off their insurance requirements.

3.

But the dilemma of board members does not stop with simple concern about the fiscal integrity of the hospital corporation. While available data indicate that relatively few doctors go without liability insurance, it is a fact that some drop their coverage because of cost or for philosophical or other considerations. Board members cannot ignore the fact that some of these physicians are highly able and qualified staff members who might move their practices to other hospitals that do not have mandatory insurance. Nor can they ignore the views of medical staff members who do not want to risk working on a case in association with an uninsured doctor and who therefore demand an insurance requirement or disclosure of the identities of their unprotected colleagues.

Hospital responses to the insurance issue have varied. Some maintain an absolute insurance requirement, others have dropped it altogether, and there is no end to the in-between approaches. They include waiver mechanisms with or without alternate financial responsibility requirements. Some require the uninsured doctors to sign indemnity agreements for the protection of other medical staff members as well as the hospital. These agreements commit uninsured physicians to pay a proportionate share of any joint judgment against them, the hospital, or other staff doctors. They also prohibit sweetheart deals with the claimant's attorney whereby uninsured doctors, to save their own economic skins, become secret allies of that lawyer in the pursuit of a judgment against the hospital or other physicians.

4.

Unlike the insurance requirement suits, which were a rarity until the cost of insurance escalated out of sight, there has been no scarcity of cases involving denials or suspension of privileges because of claimed deficiencies in credentials or competence. If a private community hospital were to be regarded as is any other private business, there would be no basis for the courts to review management decisions, regardless of how arbitrary or erroneous they appeared to be.

But hospitals, even totally private ones built without a nickel of public funds, are viewed differently. If the hospital is the only one in town, then closing the door on a physician clearly will have a devastating effect on that doctor's ability to serve patients and on the individual's economic future. Even if the hospital isn't the only one in town, a blackball at one can have a rippling effect on how a doctor is received by colleagues at other institutions. Peer review, by definition, involves a review of a doctor by peers who also may be competitors.

It is this judgment by peers, some of whom may regard their competitors (or their cronies' competitors) with less than fraternal affection, that probably prompts many judges to find a basis for reviewing such activities.

And so it is, when the hospital door is slammed on a doctor, many courts will look beyond the basic rule that such matters rest within the sound discretion of the hospital's management. They will conclude there is a right to review because of questions of monopoly, of the hospital's failure to follow its own bylaws or other rules, or of government money and regulation converting the private hospital to a quasi-public one.

When the court does review hospital staff matters, its purview ordinarily is limited. If it appears that the complaining doctor was accorded basic procedural fairness and the adverse action taken was not "arbitrary and capricious," the hospital generally will be upheld. Procedural fairness in the context of hospital staff matters does not require all the formalities of a court trial. Not infrequently, notice to the doctor of the reasons for the action taken and a fair opportunity to present the physician's witnesses and side of the case are held to be sufficient due process. If the adverse action appears to have rational relationship to the hospital's orderly operation or to advancing the interests of patients, the courts will not be inclined to stamp it as arbitrary and capricious.

Therefore Dr. Sabina's contentions about Hohokam's being the only hospital in town and its failure to follow its own medical staff bylaws gave him the key to the courthouse.

Were it not for the fact that he failed to produce any solid evidence that the suspension was the result of a conspiracy in restraint of trade, his allegations that the action was designed to suppress competition would have been troublesome. The immunities granted to peer review bodies unquestionably are broad, but a federal appeals court has ruled that such immunities do not extend to antitrust law violations.

The bottom line seems to be one of motive. If doctors and hospitals restrict, deny, or suspend privileges to reduce competition or to indulge prejudices, then judicial scrutiny is something to worry about. On the other hand, if it appears that they are earnestly looking after the interests of the patients, they will find the courts willing to follow the biblical admonition about rendering unto Caesar the things that are Caesar's. They will find the courts eager to render unto Hippocrates the things that are Hippocrates's.

Case 4

Double Trouble

PERSONAE

Judge Bertram Abel, held hearing on petition for injunction

Dr. John Brown, surgeon at Parkerstown Community Hospital, No. 2 protagonist

Dr. Walter Craft, chairman, Department of Surgery

Dr. Joseph Green, surgeon at Parkerstown, No. 1 protagonist

Lewis Hunt, president of hospital Board of Trustees

Dr. Ralph Jones, president of medical staff

Larry Larson, hospital administrator

John Lehman, hospital board member

Richard Savage, attorney for Dr. Green

Barry Seigel, attorney for hospital

Dr. Jonas Tilton, chairman of Tissue Committee

Lawrence Warren, hearing officer in the case of Dr. Green

Norman White, hospital board member

Parkerstown Community Hospital is an acute care general institution of 145 beds located in a city of 25,000. The hospital is only 10 years old and, as the only one in the area, which grew rapidly in population in the late 1950s and early 1960s, it serves the residents of the city and of the immediate surrounding townships.

The hospital was built as the result of intensive community involvement and fund raising. More than five years were consumed in the efforts to obtain money and state approvals. To develop community support for the hospital project, the organizers established a nonprofit membership corporation.

The hospital's Board of Trustees is elected from and by the membership of the corporation, one-third of the board members each year for three-year terms. Any individual 18 years or older, who lives within the hospital's service area, is eligible to become a member of the corporation upon payment of the annual $10 dues. There is no requirement of membership in the corporation for any period of time before individuals can participate in the annual election.

This corporate format helped the organizers of the hospital develop sufficient public interest, public pressure, and the support of local members of the legislature to raise the construction funds and to obtain the necessary regulatory approvals to build the hospital.

After obtaining the financing and approvals, the hospital had to overcome its next hurdle: obtaining sufficient members for its medical staff. To do this it was necessary to sell not only the opportunity of practicing in such a medical setting but also the advantages of living in a small community. The organizers understood that the success of the hospital, and its ability to repay its financing, depended upon high utilization. While local medical practitioners were happy about creation of the hospital, because it would reduce their travel time to other institutions and make practice more convenient, they alone could not generate sufficient utilization to assure financial success. They also were not particularly interested, as were the other organizers, in bringing new doctors to the community. They did not believe the city's medical needs required any substantial increase in the number of physicians. Therefore, the recruitment effort was left primarily in the hands of the nonphysician hospital leaders. The task turned out to be extremely difficult and remains a struggle to the present day.

As a result of the recruitment efforts, the board was able to attract Dr. John Brown and Dr. Joseph Green to Parkerstown. Both were recently board-certified general surgeons who came from other states. Their applications for staff membership were reviewed perfunctorily by the Credentials Committee of the medical staff and recommended to the board, which gave swift approval. The credentialing process of the medical staff and the board's appointment method were subsidiary to the recruitment operation. As one board member stated, "Once we expend the time and effort to recruit a physician, it would be ridiculous to reject him for staff appointment."

The attitude on staff appointment of many of the board members, none of whom were physicians, was simply that doctors who had the requisite education and state licensure, and particularly those who also had certification by their appropriate boards, were qualified for acceptance. One board member commented, "What else could one want after all those screening processes? Look how hard it is even to get into medical school."

* * * * *

Immediately after arriving in Parkerstown, the two physicians joined together in a professional association and opened an office directly across the street from the hospital.

For the first few months, as is the case with most new practices, Drs. Brown and Green did not receive many patients in their offices and admitted few to the hospital. However, they were personable, energetic, and interested in establishing a successful practice. They participated in many community activities and entertained local leaders as well as prominent members of the hospital corporation and of the Board of Trustees. These social efforts contributed to the growth of their practice. They exhibited a friendly concern, not only for their patients' health care but also for all their other problems. They always were available to treat patients. Individuals would visit the emergency room at night and either Dr. Brown or Dr. Green would be available to admit them and to provide care. There never was an occasion when the hospital emergency department physician on call had to come in to cover a patient of either of these doctors. As a result of this attention, their practice grew rapidly.

By the end of two years, they were admitting more patients to the hospital than any other two medical staff members. This, of course, pleased the Board of Trustees since they were contributing to utilization of the facility. However, the Tissue Committee of the medical staff started to receive a disproportionate number of reports indicating that Dr. Green was removing healthy tissue. He was called before the committee and the problem was discussed informally. As a result of this session, both the chairman of the Tissue Committee, Dr. Jonas Tilton, and the chairman of the Department of Surgery, Dr. Walter Craft, counseled Dr. Green regarding what they felt to be a lack of judgment and an excessive zeal to operate. The poor reports ceased for a while.

Six months later, the reports to the Tissue Committee again revealed excessive removals of healthy tissue. The committee arranged a new meeting with Dr. Green. At about the same time, the evening nursing supervisor and the physician/director of the emergency room met with the president of the medical staff, Dr. Ralph Jones, and the administrator, Larry Larson, to discuss Dr. Green's conduct in admitting a high number of patients through the emergency room and in performing surgery in the evening.

Both Dr. Jones and Larson, after reviewing Dr. Green's admissions through the emergency room for the previous three months, decided that most of those patients were not truly emergency cases that required immediate surgery. Dr. Jones believed that the better procedure would have been to admit these patients through normal channels, and for the surgery to have been performed during normal operating room hours. Larson urged Dr. Jones to discuss the subject with Dr. Green, emphasizing that such a practice was costly to the hospital because it involved calling people in and incurring overtime costs, as well as the fact that it was disruptive to routine operations.

Several days later Dr. Jones met with Dr. Green to discuss the issue. Without commenting upon the validity of Dr. Jones's assertion "that many of the operations truly were not emergency," Dr. Green pointed out that because of the number of operations in which he was involved and the problems he had experienced in scheduling them during normal OR hours, he had no alternative and was justified in his conduct.

The problem apparently was resolved successfully subsequently after Dr. Green met with the administrator and the director of the operating room, by providing him and Dr. Brown more OR time on a routine basis. The physicians were assured that they could start their operations at 7 A.M., three days a week, and that an operating team would be available for scheduled surgery on Saturday mornings. The doctors were pleased and the administrator envisioned higher utilization of the facilities on the weekend.

The Tissue Committee, having been apprised of the resolution of the emergency room problem, hoped that Dr. Green's conduct would improve on its own, so its planned meeting with him was not held. Healthy tissue removals dropped slightly and the committee seemed satisfied that its purpose was being accomplished. One member said: "The downward trend is a good sign and Dr. Green obviously is maturing with time and experience."

A year later the trend reversed significantly and over a three-month period, the amount of healthy tissue removal being reported increased substantially. The committee began to review the situation again.

* * * * *

At this point rumors about the review of Dr. Green's work began to travel throughout the institution. The rumors ran the gamut from his ability to practice to personal relationships. In addition, the members of the medical staff started to split into two contending factions.

One side held to the view that Dr. Green's conduct was out of the ordinary—improper—and could only result in trouble for physicians who associated themselves with him in any way. Further, the special scheduling for Drs. Green and Brown annoyed some of the older practitioners. The other faction consisted of staff members who were happy working with Dr. Green. He was always in the hospital, friendly with everyone, and appeared to keep his patients extremely happy. While the feelings of these two factions were not yet openly hostile, lines were being drawn. This was the first occasion in the hospital's brief history that such a problem had been manifested.

The Tissue Committee, upon completion of its review, concluded that Dr. Green was exhibiting poor judgment and was too eager to operate. The charts also did not contain sufficient indications to justify many of the operations he performed. The problem was discussed by Dr. Craft, the chairman of the Department of Surgery, and Dr. Jones, the president of the medical staff. They agreed that the matter should be referred to the administrator and the hospital's attorney.

* * * * *

A meeting arranged by Larson, the administrator, with the hospital's attorney, Barry Seigel, was held at the lawyer's office. All parties had felt the issue should be handled as discreetly as possible and that such a meeting, if held on the hospital's premises, would not go unnoticed by employees and staff members.

At the meeting, Dr. Jones reviewed the entire history of Dr. Green's known performance, starting with the initial problems several years before, followed by the emergency room difficulties, the additional problems with the Tissue Committee, and the current situation.

Seigel's initial advice to the administrator and to Dr. Jones, consistent with what he perceived to be the attitude of the Board of Trustees, was that they attempt to determine whether the case could be worked out amicably. He was aware of the board's reluctance to stir up a battle with a "census builder." Dr. Jones objected to this approach on the grounds that such attempts had been made in the past and that it appeared Dr. Green was going to continue to backslide unless confronted either with severe disciplinary action that would change his approach fundamentally or full revocation of his staff appointment.

Seigel then took another tack. He suggested that, before any action was taken, the problem should be reviewed by an outside medical consultant. "This course of involving an outsider," he said, "would provide objectivity because the opinion of an expert who had no personal relationships or economic stake in the outcome would not be subject to an attack questioning motivation if fault is found with Dr. Green's work."

This satisfied Dr. Jones since he assumed that any reputable reviewer would confirm the findings of the Tissue Committee. Larson, the administrator, was pleased since the delay that would result from the time needed to find a consultant and obtain a report would avoid an immediate confrontation with Dr. Green, overt involvement with the medical staff, and a possible struggle with the Board of Trustees. He believed that, if an independent consultant provided substantial support for Dr. Jones's position, the medical staff president would be in a better position to discuss the problem with the board. He hoped that when confronted with the consultant's report, Dr. Green would agree to an amicable resolution of the problem. The administrator never ignored for long the fact that Dr. Green and his partner used the hospital heavily and that the board considered this very important.

A consultant who was a faculty member at a school of medicine in another state was selected to review Dr. Green's charts. Dr. Jones chose what he believed were the most damaging ones, and a meeting was arranged outside of the hospital for the consultant to review them.

The consultant's report confirmed that Dr. Green indeed often lacked sound judgment and frequently operated when the medical indications did not support such a decision. With this preliminary report in hand, Dr. Jones recommended to Larson that the consultant review all of the charts that had formed the basis of the Tissue Committee's recommendation. The administrator then discussed this proposal with the hospital's attorney, who suggested that, before any further review, the matter be discussed with the president of the Board of Trustees, Lewis Hunt.

Seigel, Larson, and Hunt met for dinner a few evenings later. Larson recounted, primarily for Hunt's benefit, the problems with Dr. Green uncovered by the Tissue Committee, other difficulties with him, and the substance of the consultant's report. Hunt appeared deeply concerned, if not shocked, by what he heard.

"We have never had such problem at the hospital," Hunt said and then, turning to look at Larson directly, added, "have we?"

After a pause, he went on:

"When we recruited Dr. Green, I thought he was a real find. Perhaps we should have wondered why he was willing to leave Ohio, or Indiana, or wherever. He is an accepted member of the community now. He's well-liked and he certainly helps fill the hospital. Bad publicity could kill the hospital. What should we do?"

Larson looked over to Seigel, "Can we find a way to make the problem go away?"

Seigel shrugged, then said, "This is a problem that could only continue to haunt the hospital. Something must be done. The best thing to do is to have the consultant complete the investigation, and then we can best determine what the hospital can do. A meeting could be held with Dr. Green after the facts are in at which time a satisfactory resolution might be achieved."

Seigel then gave Hunt a lecture about the expanding responsibilities of hospital boards, administrators, and medical staffs to regulate their physicians for the protection of the public. He outlined problems at other institutions and spared few details of the Dr. Nork incident in California, involving a drug-using surgeon who performed unnecessary procedures with disastrous results for his patients. He cautioned Hunt and Larson that the hospital was in what he termed a "no-win" situation.

"If we take action against Dr. Green and it becomes generally known that he practiced bad medicine, operating when operations were not called for, and had other failings, then the hospital might be subject to suits for allowing malpractice or unnecessary surgery," Seigel said. "But if we ignore his performance, later we could have even more liability exposure."

He agreed that an attempt should be made to find a quiet resolution of the problem, but he was not optimistic.

As a result of this meeting, Larson, as administrator, authorized the consultant to complete his investigation. The consultant confirmed the findings of the Tissue Committee right down the line. The final report was discussed by Hunt and Larson, and they held another meeting with Seigel. No one had even mentioned letting Dr. Jones, the president of the medical staff, know where the matter stood at this point until Larson suggested dinner with him and Dr. Green to try to settle the problem. Hunt liked the proposal; Seigel expressed doubts, but went along. Larson left to give Dr. Jones an update on the situation.

* * * * *

The dinner was held at Dr. Jones's home and the three, after a wooden exchange of trivia—sports, local politics, and the like—got down to the real business at hand. Dr. Jones took the lead, reporting the results of the outside study and the risk of liability to which Dr. Green was exposing not only himself but the hospital as well. Hunt continually interjected that he and his Board of Trustees wanted to resolve the matter in a way that would not be injurious to Dr. Green but would result in avoiding any future problems.

Dr. Green listened patiently. When his turn came, the dam burst. He vigorously denied that his performance was substandard. He said he felt he was being persecuted. He pointed out that he was younger than many members of the medical staff, that he had not grown up in the area, and that he was not a member of the medical community that had been around when the hospital was established.

"My partner and I do a lot of work," he said, "we work harder than most of the other docs. They resent us."

He said he believed he was being singled out.

"Sure, I'll talk with you," Dr. Green continued, "but the board, Larson, and an attorney, aren't competent to pass upon the way I practice medicine. Your consultant, whose name you haven't even told me, probably is a faculty hack. And you," he said directly to Dr. Jones, "have always had it in for me."

He declared that the medical staff, while technically competent to pass upon his practice, was resentful of his success and therefore could not judge objectively. He suggested, as a first step at this juncture, that a consultant of his choosing be retained at the hospital's expense to look at the charts and to comment. Dr. Jones, the medical staff president, rejected this approach vigorously. But Hunt said he would consider it and would get back to both Dr. Green and Dr. Jones. The meeting ended with Dr. Jones angry at Hunt as president of the Board of Trustees for not backing him up, with Dr. Green angry at Dr. Jones and Hunt, and with Hunt believing he needed some advice.

Hunt telephoned Seigel and related what had occurred. The attorney suggested it might be possible to get the two doctors to agree to search for a jointly acceptable expert to review the files. Hunt conveyed this thought to both Drs. Jones and Green. Neither rejected it outright but expressed little enthusiasm for the proposal. Both knew that it was very unlikely they would agree on a consultant.

* * * * *

It was now December of 1977, time for the election of a third of the hospital board at the membership's annual meeting. As yet there never had been a contested vote. The election usually was secondary to a buffet dinner and dance. The meeting also had served as a fund-raising event for the hospital. Dr. Green and his partner began urging their patients to join the hospital corporation, if they hadn't already. They suggested that, as members of the public participating in the corporation, they could support the hospital and participate in selecting the trustees. A considerable number of patients and their family members took the advice.

At the annual meeting, the Nominating Committee submitted its slate of five nominees for the board. Five other individuals, all recognized as friendly to Dr. Green, were nominated from the floor. The vote resulted in the replacement of three incumbents by three supporters of Dr. Green and his partner. The board held its annual organization meeting the following week and Hunt was re-elected president, but not unanimously.

* * * * *

Rumors and gossips about Dr. Green, which already had begun to circulate, grew in scope and volume. The administrator was becoming more and more troubled and felt the matter could not drag on forever. However, Larson could see there was no effective method of confronting the problem without creating open controversy.

The proposal for a jointly selected consultant apparently had died without being rejected outright by either Dr. Green or Dr. Jones. Larson then decided to impose that procedure upon Dr. Jones, and to find out whether he could get Dr. Green to agree. Various physicians were proposed, none of whom were acceptable to Dr. Green, who then submitted a list of names, none of which were acceptable to Jones. The hospital's attorney recommended to Larson that they be rejected, and the advice was accepted.

During this period Dr. Green's conduct did not improve. The Tissue Committee continued to report that an excessive amount of healthy tissue was being removed. His emergency room admissions continued to increase, as did the night surgery. Dr. Green's conduct had become well known to the members of the medical staff and was raising questions in the minds of many physicians, the most prominent being whether they wanted to be involved in the care of any patient of Dr. Green or his partner.

* * * * *

In the absence of action by anyone else, the chairman of the Department of Surgery, Dr. Craft, after reviewing the consultant's report and the charts he relied upon, and some additional charts of patients treated since that report, made a formal recommendation that Dr. Green's privileges be revoked under the medical staff bylaws. His recommendation was received and reviewed by the Executive Committee of the medical staff, which voted to initiate procedures for revocation of Dr. Green's staff appointment.

The president of the Board of Trustees, Hunt, was furious. The medical staff had taken a position overtly and publicly against Dr. Green, thereby foreclosing any further opportunities for a quiet settlement. He met with the hospital's attorney, Seigel, who advised him that the only path available now was to avoid interfering with the medical staff's actions and to permit the matter to go to a hearing in accordance with the staff bylaws.

Dr. Green, upon receipt of the charges, promptly retained an attorney, Richard Savage, who immediately filed suit in state court to enjoin the hospital and the Board of Trustees from proceeding under the bylaws. Judge Bertram Abel, upon receiving notice from Dr. Green's attorney, directed that he contact the hospital's attorney. Savage telephoned Seigel and gave him the outline of the allegations, the relief sought, and the time of the hearing before the judge.

The medical staff bylaws provided that, if any adverse action was recommended against a physician, the doctor would be entitled to a hearing before the hospital's Credentials Committee. The bylaws also stated that that committee should be composed of the heads of all of the medical staff departments. These chairmen also served as members of the medical staff's Executive Committee, along with several other physicians.

Not surprisingly, Savage told Seigel the first ground for Dr. Green's challenge was that the members of the Credentials Committee, who would serve as the hearing panel, already had passed upon the allegations against him in their capacities as members of the Executive Committee. In addition, Savage asserted that any part of the medical staff was an inappropriate forum for the hearing and that the matter should be resolved by the courts. He also contended that the charges were not supported by sufficient evidence and were being pressed to harass Dr. Green as part of a conspiracy among members of the medical staff to deny him his right to practice, in violation of antitrust law. Finally, Savage intimated that he might join every physician on the medical staff as a defendant.

As soon as he finished talking with Savage, Seigel, in a conference call, advised Hunt and Larson that litigation was under way and sought their views on the hospital's response. They asked Seigel for his plan for action. He told them he could block court action seeking to enjoin the hospital from proceeding according to the bylaws but he urged that the hearing process be commenced as soon as possible.

Hunt then asked several questions: Could Seigel assist in the presentation of the case against Dr. Green and also advise the board? Who actually would present the case against Dr. Green before the Credentials Committee? How much was this whole thing going to cost?

Seigel addressed the cost question first, telling Hunt and Larson that "big dollars" were involved and adding that it "is a cost of doing business" that "can't be avoided without possibly greater expenses later." He told them that a physician was needed to present the case against Dr. Green and that if he, Seigel, played a major role in assisting in this effort, it would present problems in his advising the board later on its decision on revocation of, or other action in respect to, the appointment.

They then turned to the hearing procedures. The medical staff bylaws called for a hearing officer but did not require that individual to be an attorney. The bylaws were silent on whether Dr. Green could be assisted by an attorney at the hearing. Hunt asked whether Dr. Green should be permitted to have a lawyer present.

"The trend of cases today, in 1978, suggests that one of these days soon a court will say due process for a doctor requires participation of counsel at a hearing," Seigel replied. "Frankly, I would hate to deny counsel and run the risk that the state supreme court, after we had a hearing and it went to court, would find a denial of fairness and require us to start all over because we didn't allow Dr. Green an attorney."

"All right, let him have a lawyer," the board president said. "It's going to cost him money if he fights us. Let's make him spend like we'll have to spend."

"Don't worry about him spending dollars," Seigel responded. "Savage doesn't work for peanuts. He probably has $5,000 up front already. We also need a hearing officer, who would advise the medical staff Credentials Committee, and he should be an attorney. We need the attorney to assure an adequate record, to avoid partiality, and to minimize error at the hearing. A physician might be intimidated by an attorney. Actually, if the hearing officer is an attorney, and Dr. Green is represented by an attorney, the case against the doctor most probably could be presented effectively only by an attorney, not a medical staff member, as we decided a while ago."

This disturbed both Larson and Hunt, who expressed the view that the matter was becoming "much too legalistic," but they accepted Seigel's recommendation.

They focused next on the legal proceeding Dr. Green had instituted and agreed that Seigel should go to court representing both the medical staff and the hospital, at least at this time, and they would cross the bridge of separate counsel after they saw what happened there.

* * * * *

Seigel and Savage appeared before Judge Abel the next day on the motion for a preliminary injunction. The judge suggested that the attorneys meet with him in chambers to discuss the nature of the action and to determine whether the parties could reach a settlement. Judge Abel, as a resident of the community, was very familiar with the hospital and was hopeful the matter could be resolved.

In chambers, Seigel set forth the background of the case and informed Judge Abel that the hospital was ready to provide Dr. Green with a hearing to which he was entitled under the bylaws. Savage objected on the grounds that the members of the hearing committee already had made up their mind regarding his client and that that committee could not be impartial under any circumstances. Not only were the members of the Credentials Committee, which would serve as the hearing panel, on the Executive Committee, Savage declared, but many medical staff members had been exposed, through rumor, to the alleged incidents that formed the basis of the adverse recommendation.

The judge pondered the question. While working his way to an answer, he frequently made remarks such as, "Nobody wants the hospital to get hurt," and finally suggested that the matter be resolved by an ad hoc hearing committee consisting of members of the medical staff who were not members of the Executive Committee.

The judge said he understood and agreed with the position of Dr. Green's attorney generally but felt that the medical staff was the appropriate body to hear the case and to make a recommendation to the board. He said, much to Seigel's chagrin, "There will be ample opportunity for judicial review upon completion of the hearing and action by the board."

Seigel told Judge Abel, "I'm afraid that your remark is a signal to Dr. Green that no matter how well we handle the hearing, he should come back to court."

Savage rejoined, "In America, freedom is protected by the courts."

The judge told both attorneys to calm down.

Seigel then requested, in light of the fact that the hearing would not be conducted pursuant to the bylaws, that Judge Abel issue an order to that effect, and he agreed. The order directed that a hearing be held by an ad hoc committee of the medical staff that could not include any members who had been involved previously in passing upon the recommendation, or who would testify.

* * * * *

After the court proceeding ended, Seigel reviewed the law on medical staff hearings and concluded that the session had better be conducted like a trial. He therefore recommended to Hunt and Larson that he be authorized to retain the services of another attorney to serve as the hearing officer, and that he, Seigel, present the case on behalf of the medical staff. He told them a court reporter should be retained to take and transcribe the testimony.

The board president and administrator, with Dr. Jones, the medical staff president, then reviewed the list of staff physicians and, in line with the court order, selected as candidates for the ad hoc committee a number of the more mature members who had not been involved in the process thus far. Dr. Jones accepted the responsibility for contacting the physicians and appointing them to the committee.

The next day Seigel contacted Savage, Dr. Green's attorney, and explained the procedure the medical staff intended to follow. Savage complained about the method for selecting the members of the ad hoc committee, even though he did not have specific objections to any of the individuals who had agreed to serve and had been appointed. Most had agreed with considerable reluctance and only after a "selling job" by Dr. Jones. They were most concerned about the time they would have to devote to the hearing.

Seigel decided that Lawrence Warren, with whom he had attended law school and who was a magistrate in a neighboring community, would be an appropriate individual to serve as the hearing officer. He contacted Warren and obtained his agreement to participate on an hourly fee basis.

Larson had the chore of setting up the hearing at a time convenient to the witnesses, Dr. Green, the members of the hearing committee, the hearing officer, and the attorneys. This task turned out to be more time consuming than anyone imagined; it took Larson almost a week to arrange a date on which all parties would be available. Meanwhile, Seigel reviewed all of the records that had formed the basis of the various recommendations of the Tissue Committee, as well as the data of the Emergency Room Committee. He met with the consultant and they spent much time on his report and his proposed testimony.

* * * * *

A regular meeting of the board happened to occur before the hearing was to be held. At the meeting Hunt, as board president, reported on the activities of the medical staff as they related to Dr. Green, the events before Judge Abel—about which nothing had appeared in the local press—and the fact that a hearing would be conducted.

John Lehman, a board member known as a supporter of Dr. Green, immediately questioned Hunt as to the reasons and motives for the medical staff activities directed against Dr. Green. He said he felt Dr. Green was being singled out by the older members of the medical community, not for professional reasons but because of his success.

Lehman made a motion, which was seconded, that a special ad hoc committee of the board be appointed to investigate the activities of the medical staff, particularly of those members who had been involved in preferring the charges against Dr. Green. He stated his belief that the leadership of the medical staff—members of the Tissue Committee and the Executive Committee in particular—had not contributed to the hospital to the extent that Dr. Green and his partner had. Therefore, Lehman said, it was in the interest of the board to see that Dr. Green was not being "persecuted" and that he receive a fair hearing.

Another board member, Norman White, who had recruited Dr. Green and was still a member of the hospital's Physician Recruitment Committee, expressed concern about the impact the proceeding would have on the ability to attract other young physicians. He traced the history of the recruiting problems his committee had experienced, the contributions of Dr. Green and his partner to the utilization of the hospital, and the continuing difficulty in finding physicians to join the staff. He said his feelings were ambivalent.

"Specifically," White said, "I am opposed to physicians who are not providing good health care but, at the same time, I am not sure that Dr. Green is guilty of such charges and these proceedings are just going to create an adverse situation for the hospital."

Hunt pointed out that no decision had to be made by the board at this time, and that since a hearing was to be held at which Dr. Green could tell his side, an investigation by the board was not in order. There followed a general discussion that indicated to Hunt that the members had a great lack of understanding about the board's responsibilities.

Hunt then suggested that the board hold a special meeting at which the hospital's attorney, Seigel, would explain in detail what had occurred and why the hospital was taking the steps it was taking. There was general agreement with the recommendation and Lehman's motion for an ad hoc committee to investigate the medical staff was tabled by unanimous vote.

The following Monday night the special meeting was held. Seigel explained all of the events that had led up to the hearing, as well as related developments in the law that were occurring throughout the country. He emphasized not only the rights of Dr. Green to a hearing but also the obligations of the medical staff and the hospital to the public.

Many board members were upset to learn of their possible liability exposure and expressed their concern. They felt they had not been briefed adequately on their personal liability when they became members and wanted assurances from the hospital against any lawsuits based on alleged failures on their part. Seigel assured them he would look into the questions they raised and would discuss with the hospital's insurance agent the extent of their protection and, if it was not adequate, whether it could be obtained. No one sought to bring to a vote Lehman's motion, which had been tabled at the previous meeting, for a board committee to investigate the medical staff.

Later that evening Larson, the administrator, who had attended the board meeting, answered an advertisement in a hospital journal about a position as chief executive officer at an institution in another state.

* * * * *

Warren, the designated hearing officer, arranged to meet with the members of the hearing committee before the session to discuss in detail how the proceeding would be conducted. The physicians were less concerned with the procedures than with their liability exposure as a result of serving on the hearing panel. Warren assured them they "could not be sued as a result of being members of the hearing committee'' so long as they participated in good faith and reached a decision that was supported by the evidence presented to them. With this advice the members felt fairly secure in performing their duties.

Warren viewed the hearing as no different from a trial, and he had presided over many as a magistrate. As he saw it, his role would be that of a judge, and the role of the committee that of a jury.

The hearing was to be held from 7 to 11 P.M., beginning on a Monday, with Tuesday and Wednesday nights available if needed. However, Seigel and Savage already had estimated it would take four to five nights to present all of the evidence.

The hospital auditorium was chosen for the hearing. Seigel, on arriving, found the auditorium occupied not only with witnesses but also with many patients and friends of Dr. Green. Seigel feared that Dr. Green intended to try to intimidate the hearing committee and the witnesses. He requested a conference with Warren and Savage, at which he asked Warren to recess the hearing and reconvene it in a smaller room, limited solely to the members of the hearing committee, Dr. Green and his attorney, and the witnesses. Savage objected, saying that Dr. Green was entitled to a public hearing if he so desired. After further discussion, Warren recessed the proceeding for that evening.

The next morning he contacted both attorneys and informed them he would limit attendance solely to the members of the hearing committee, Dr. Green and his attorney, Seigel, and the witnesses. Savage again objected, threatening to go back to court, but Warren maintained his position and the attorney gave in.

That evening the hearing was convened in the medical staff library. The first order of business was Savage's objections to Warren as the hearing officer as well as to the members of the hearing committee on the ground that, as members of the medical staff, they were not impartial. Warren overruled the objections and directed Seigel to proceed with the case.

The first witness was Dr. Tilton, chairman of the Tissue Committee. He reviewed the history of Dr. Green's involvement with that committee. All of the charts that had formed the basis of the committee's various recommendations were introduced and discussed. When given the opportunity, Savage questioned Dr. Tilton closely about his working relationship with Dr. Green and any possible personality conflicts between them. Savage's theme was that Dr. Tilton was using the Tissue Committee to ''get even'' with Dr. Green. The witness steadfastly refused to agree that this was the case at all. The testimony and cross-examination consumed so much time that the hearing was recessed for the night after only the one witness had testified.

The next morning, a front-page article in the *Parkerstown Courier,* the local newspaper, said a hearing at the hospital was being conducted in private over the objections of Dr. Green, who felt the public should participate. The article also said the board had been asked to form a committee to investigate the members of the medical staff who were involved in preferring charges against Dr. Green. The newspaper did not attribute its report to any specific sources.

Hunt, the board president, was furious and directed Larson to determine how the information reached the newspaper. The editor refused to disclose his sources but requested a statement from the hospital regarding the activities of Dr. Green, the medical staff, and the board. Larson discussed the matter with Seigel and Hunt and told the editor:

"In light of the hearing, the hospital does not believe that it could comment at this time. Dr. Green will be given an opportunity to tell his story, and the hospital can assure the public that all physicians are treated fairly and that the public interest is being protected."

The next session heard testimony by the director of the emergency room and the evening nursing supervisor as to Dr. Green's activities in emergency and in the evening operations. This direct testimony, and Savage's cross-examination, which followed the line of his questioning of the chairman of the Tissue Committee, consumed the entire evening.

On the weekend another newspaper article appeared on the activities of the hearing committee, as well as an editorial suggesting the entire conduct of the medical staff be subject to scrutiny. The editorial took exception to the closed nature of Dr. Green's hearing.

The following week the hearings resumed with the testimony of the consultant. On direct examination he reviewed the charts and gave his opinion, with reasons, regarding the lack of necessity for the surgery for the patients covered by those charts. Savage briefly reviewed the consultant's background and pressed the points that the expert had been retained initially on the recommendation of Dr. Jones, the president of the medical staff, was being "paid for his testimony," and that Dr. Jones had reviewed the charts with him. However, he was unable to shake the consultant's opinion regarding the surgery Dr. Green performed. Upon completion of the cross-examination, Savage requested a week's recess so he could adequately prepare Dr. Green's case. Warren and the members of the hearing committee agreed and a date as set in the following week.

* * * * *

During this interval in the hearing, Larson received a telephone call from the Inspector General's office in the Department of Health, Education, and Welfare, regarding Dr. Green's activities. DHEW asked to meet with Larson to discuss Dr. Green and to review his charts. The administrator offered to call back. He immediately set up a conference call with Seigel and Hunt and reported on the DHEW contact. Hunt was practically distraught.

"When I signed on to be president of the board I never expected all this turmoil and trouble," he complained. "I have my own business to run. You both get paid for what you do, I don't. We should have settled the matter with Dr. Green quietly and the medical staff should not have gone off on its own with the charges. Now the hospital is going to have to deal with the feds. It's terrible."

Seigel expressed sympathy but pointed out that the hospital had no alternative but to meet, and cooperate, with DHEW, and to continue the hearing. After much discussion they all agreed. They also decided not to inform Dr. Green or his attorney about the DHEW interest at this point.

* * * * *

When the hearing reconvened, Dr. Green took the stand and on direct testimony described his personal problems with the members of the Tissue Committee and the Executive Committee. He stated several times that the members were "out to get him." The charges against him were not based upon any solid medical evidence, he asserted, but solely upon personality differences.

"Who better than I knows the facts regarding each patient?" he asked. "They are jealous of me because I have become the most successful surgeon in the community."

On cross-examination, when confronted with the charts, his response repeatedly was "in my opinion the operation was necessary." He further emphasized that he was a board-certified surgeon and that his training provided him with the ability to make the decisions that now were being questioned. He expressed the view that the members of the ad hoc committee, none of whom was a board-certified surgeon, were not capable of passing upon his judgments on the need for surgery.

The next evening another consultant testified on behalf of Dr. Green that he had reviewed the charts and felt there was no indication of unnecessary surgery. He steadfastly maintained his position under intense cross-examination.

After completion of the testimony, both attorneys summarized the evidence that had been presented. The hearing then was recessed. The following evening the hearing committee met with Warren. They reviewed all of the documentary evidence presented and decided upon their recommendations. Meanwhile, the newspaper submitted questions to Larson seeking to ascertain what had occurred at the hearing but the administrator did not respond. Larson sent résumés to two more hospitals' search committees.

The hearing committee report, signed by all of its members, recommended that Dr. Green's privileges and staff appointment be revoked. It stated that the charts, as testified to by the witnesses on behalf of the medical staff, indicated a serious lack of judgment in the performance of operations that were not necessary, and cited violations of procedures for scheduling surgery. Larson forwarded the report to both attorneys and to Hunt. Savage promptly contacted Hunt and requested the opportunity to appear with his client before the board. After consultation with Seigel, Hunt agreed even though the medical staff bylaws did not require such a meeting at this time and Judge Abel had not ordered such a procedure.

At that special board meeting, Savage requested that a full hearing be scheduled before the trustees on the charges against his client. He argued that the hearing before the medical staff panel could not be considered valid since it was conducted by staff members who were prejudiced against Dr. Green. Seigel reviewed the law as he saw it, as well as the procedure usually followed at other hospitals, and argued that the board should review the hearing transcript but should not grant Dr. Green a de novo hearing before the trustees. The attorneys and Dr. Green then were excused by Hunt and a bitter debate followed over the procedure the board should follow.

By a close vote it was decided the review would be on the record and that a new hearing would not be conducted before the board. Hunt then directed Seigel to obtain the transcript of the hearing for the board's review as soon as possible. When the transcript was completed, copies were distributed to all board members. Another special board meeting was scheduled to discuss the evidence and to hear final arguments from Dr. Green's attorney and Seigel.

Without consulting with anyone, Hunt decided to take one last shot at attempting to resolve the dispute. The board president met with Savage and proposed a settlement whereby Dr. Green would agree either to resign or to gradually leave the hospital. Hunt believed both of these courses would be acceptable to the medical staff. Dr. Green's attorney summarily rejected the proposal.

* * * * *

At the board meeting, after much debate it was decided to modify the recommendations of the hearing committee to the extent that Dr. Green would be placed on restricted privileges under supervision of Dr. Craft, the chairman of the Department of Surgery. He could perform no surgery without a concurring opinion, either from the chairman or from a surgeon designated by him. Hunt believed this resolution of the problem, which he lobbied for strenuously, would be a workable compromise, acceptable to both the medical staff and to Dr. Green. The vote was 10 to 5 in favor of this proposal.

The next day, Seigel received a call from Dr. Green's attorney stating that he was going before Judge Abel to obtain an injunction against the enforcement of the decision and to seek other relief. Upon arriving in Judge Abel's chambers Seigel was handed a new complaint and an order to show cause that, to his shock and dismay, named him, along with the members of the board who had voted in favor of the decision on Dr. Green; the members of the hearing committee; Warren, the hearing officer; Larson; Dr. Jones, the president of the medical staff; the hospital; the medical staff; the named members of the Tissue Committee and the Emergency Room Committee; several nurses, and the hospital's medical consultant, as defendants. It sought $5 million in damages for violating the state antitrust laws, state conspiracy laws, and torts including interference with a contractual relationship.

As soon as he could, Seigel told Judge Abel that since he now was named a defendant, it would be inappropriate for him to appear on behalf of anyone other than himself. Judge Abel agreed but suggested that, for a few brief moments, the parties attempt to discuss a settlement with him. The judge indicated that, without passing upon the merits, he felt the board's decision was the basis for a compromise and that possibly it could be slightly modified to be made acceptable to Dr. Green.

Savage refused to discuss compromise. He wanted the entire decision overturned and his client to be permitted to continue to practice without interference by the medical staff. In light of this, Judge Abel postponed any determination on the order to show cause, to give the parties the opportunity to obtain counsel.

During the next several days everyone obtained attorneys. Physicians who were specifically named looked to their insurance companies' attorneys under their malpractice policies. The hospital was represented by its insurance company counsel on the damages issues but was required to obtain another attorney to represent it on the equitable relief sought. This attorney represented both the hospital and the medical staff on this issue. However, none of the insurance companies would defend the medical staff on the damage claims since it was asserted they were not "covered" by any policy. Hunt, at Seigel's suggestion, authorized the attorney appearing on behalf of the hospital to represent the medical staff.

When Judge Abel convened a hearing of counsel for all of the parties, he jokingly commented that this was a meeting of the Parkerstown bar, with many guests from other communities in the county. After hearing argument from Savage, Dr. Green's attorney, the judge declined to issue an injunction. With respect to the complaint itself, he directed the attorneys to work out a discovery schedule and a motion schedule so the case could be resolved expeditiously.

The following day the local newspaper had a major front-page article about the lawsuit and the day after that some of Dr. Green's patients picketed the hospital with signs accusing it of discriminating against him.

* * * * *

Meanwhile, DHEW had begun its investigation into Dr. Green's performance. The hospital learned that DHEW believed Dr. Green was involved in questionable operations and that his partner, Dr. Brown, also was probably guilty of the same failings. Larson passed this information on to Hunt, Dr. Jones, and Seigel. After some discussion Larson proposed that a review of Dr. Brown's charts be undertaken quietly, and they all agreed to this course, although Hunt expressed misgivings.

Dr. Jones, as president of the medical staff, personally reviewed a number of Dr. Brown's charts and, while no one indicated outrageous conduct, in his opinion they showed a pattern of questionable activities. Before any decisions were reached about what to do with these findings, DHEW requested a meeting with hospital representatives regarding the conduct of both Dr. Green and Dr. Brown. Larson and Dr. Jones told Hunt that they could not sit by regarding Dr. Brown, since his activity at the institution was a subject of investigation by DHEW.

Dr. Jones directed the Tissue Committee to review Dr. Brown's charts. The committee members objected on the ground that they would be subject to another suit. However, after much cajoling, Dr. Brown's charts were reviewed. The chairman of the Tissue Committee reported finding a pattern similar to that of Dr. Green. Then, before completing the review, a majority of the Tissue Committee members resigned, expressing fear of being sued if they made any adverse recommendations about Dr. Brown. Dr. Jones sought and received board permission to retain an outside consultant other than the one who had reviewed Dr. Green's charts. This consultant's review confirmed the doubts regarding Dr. Brown.

Dr. Jones recommended to the Executive Committee that Dr. Brown's conduct be referred to an ad hoc hearing committee, to avoid the difficulty that had become evident in Dr. Green's situation. The medical staff bylaws had not been modified to conform to the court's ruling that the Credentials Committee was not an appropriate forum. The matter was deferred until the Executive Committee could meet with Seigel to obtain guidance.

At that meeting Seigel agreed Dr. Brown's case should be referred to an ad hoc hearing committee. When Dr. Jones attempted to appoint such a panel, no member of the staff could be found who was willing to serve. They refused on the basis that they were being sued by Dr. Brown's partner, Dr. Green, and believed that they could not serve impartially. They also were reluctant to run the risk of being sued by Dr. Brown because they had few doubts that he would do so if they participated in proceedings that resulted in adverse action against him.

Meanwhile, Seigel could not find another attorney who was willing to serve as the hearing officer. It was well known that Warren, who had been the first hearing officer, was now a defendant and was forced to incur the expenses of defending himself as a conspirator, although the hospital had indicated it probably would indemnify him and reimburse him for his expenses.

Confronted with these difficulties, Hunt convened a board meeting to discuss Dr. Brown's situation. The board was reluctant to get involved at all with Dr. Brown. However, the members realized the hospital might have problems with DHEW if they did not act against him. The board directed Larson, the administrator, to confer with Dr. Jones to attempt to find a way to get members of the medical staff to participate.

After much discussion among Larson, physicians on the medical staff, and Seigel, a proposal was drafted for the board to adopt a resolution to defend and to indemnify the medical staff members for their participation in good faith in peer review proceedings, in the event of litigation. When this motion was presented, one board member, John Lehman, objected, as he had in the Green case. He contended that the medical staff would rely upon protection by indemnification to continue its "persecution" of certain members of the staff, and he urged defeat of the resolution.

However, it was passed, with the modification that it would apply not only to the members of the medical staff but also to the board. With this resolution in hand, Seigel met with members of the medical staff and gave his opinion that they had little exposure. They disagreed, and some referred to Warren's earlier statement to the hearing committee. As one put it, "Why believe anything an attorney says?"

Therefore, even with the resolution, Dr. Jones was unable to obtain staff members to serve on the ad hoc hearing committee. Very distressed, he then appointed several senior staff members to the hearing panel without their agreement to serve. Meanwhile, Seigel, confronted with the problem of finding a hearing officer, obtained one only after the Board of Trustees passed another indemnification resolution applicable to him.

With these procedural difficulties possibly overcome, Larson notified Dr. Brown of the charges and of proposed hearing dates. Savage, who also was now Dr. Brown's attorney, objected to the proposed members of the ad hoc hearing committee. Upon learning of this, all the members enthusiastically agreed with the objections and excused themselves from participating. Dr. Jones and Seigel realized there was no way they were going to obtain a hearing committee within the hospital.

Seigel then went to court, seeking to have Judge Abel determine the manner in which the hearing on Dr. Brown's conduct should be conducted. At a session in chambers with only the attorneys present, Judge Abel expressed his disgust at the entire situation at the hospital. He said it was a disgrace to the community and a benefit to no one.

Acknowledging that he could not pass upon the merits regarding either Dr. Green or Dr. Brown at the time, and that he could understand the reluctance of the medical staff members to participate, he declared that the institution was obliged to provide Dr. Brown with a hearing within the hospital setting. He made no rulings, saying he would take the matter under advisement, but expressed clearly to both attorneys his view that the court should not be the forum at this stage. He directed the attorneys to attempt to find a panel of physicians who would serve as the ad hoc hearing committee. He also requested them to submit memoranda on the limited issue of the scope of judicial review after a board decision based on a hearing recommendation. He pointed out that these were "legal questions." With this accomplished, he sent the attorneys on their way.

Seigel considered himself to be in an unenviable situation. He had no plan for forming a hearing committee from the medical staff, he was a defendant in Dr. Green's case but still advising the hospital regarding that physician, he was expected to deal with DHEW in the investigations of Drs. Green and Brown, and he was hearing rumblings of possible malpractice litigation against the two in which the hospital might be joined. It was evident that Dr. Brown and Dr. Green were not going to bow out graciously but intended to cause protracted litigation, and the hospital's legal and hearing costs already were substantial.

When Seigel reported to Hunt on the then current situation, the board president told the attorney that, "We should have settled the matter quietly as I suggested." Seigel was bewildered by the comment and saw no way to restore the hospital to a normal situation.

Commentary

1.

The usual reluctance to commence formal proceedings against a medical staff member was increased by the high utilization of the hospital by the physician in question. While it is a matter of conjecture, prompt instituting of the formal disciplinary procedures against Dr. Green might have resulted either in permanent improvement on his part or, if that did not occur, in his removal from the staff before he had fully entrenched himself in the community and built such a large practice, thus avoiding the turmoil he had created.

More frequently than is believed by the public and hospital critics, medical staff leadership is more aggressive in seeking to discipline a physician than are hospital boards. Here, Hunt, the board president, sought a peaceful, quiet way out, which may have compounded the problem in that he left Dr. Jones, the president of the medical staff, and Dr. Craft, the surgery department chairman, out on a limb. It is noteworthy that even after the hearing, with all the travail it entailed, the board, led by Hunt, still looked for a "compromise."

2.

In recruiting, a hospital should be wary of physicians with excellent paper credentials who are easily enticed into relocating. As part of the recruiting process, the usual review of qualifications, behavior, and past professional performance that attends initial appointment should be very thorough. Dr. Green's past record might have revealed reasons why he was not a choice recruit.

3.

The prospects for getting out of the disciplinary process morass at Parkerstown Community Hospital were not good. Experience indicates that the first disciplinary proceeding at a hospital often sets the tone for those that follow. Lack of success in one leads to increased reluctance to invoke discipline later.

The board members were not well aware of their responsibilities, particularly in disciplinary cases, which is as much a fault of administration as of the board itself. Educational programs for board members are on the increase and many deal with board-staff relationships, liability exposure, indemnification practices, and other matters that arose in the case study.

4.

Democracy and public participation in hospital affairs are positive values in society. Yet the election of board members by the membership of a corporation or a hospital association poses danger. When a struggle occurs between the medical staff and the board, or between a physician and the hospital, attempts may be undertaken to change the balance of power by changing the board's composition through the election process.

To prevent what may well be sudden, violent upheavals at hospitals with board election processes, several techniques can be used. One, illustrated in the case study, is to allow no more than one-third of the board seats to be filled by election in a single year. A second is to provide in the bylaws that no one is eligible to vote in an election of board members who has not been a member for at least 60, or even 90, days. In addition, the corporate secretary, the administrator, or some other official of the corporation or hospital should review regularly the changes in the corporate or association membership to detect trends that may indicate a movement to bring substantial change to the hospital.

Attempts to stack a hospital corporation or association membership often are not brought about by basic policy or philosophy differences but, rather, have a single purpose, such as protection of a physician on the staff or the removal of the hospital's chief executive. They are similar to single-issue politics, which is discernably on the increase across the country.

5.

The medical staff is entitled to know of the legal and other safeguards provided to its members who participate actively in peer review activities. Failure to provide complete and accurate information about the applicable legal rules of the jurisdiction, both statutory and judicially created, insurance protection, and the policy of the hospital as to indemnification and payment of legal expenses of medical staff members, can only lead to lack of confidence on the part of the staff when difficulties arise.

In the case study, Warren, the magistrate who conducted the hearing, was not the proper person to provide information to the members of the hearing committee. His failure to distinguish clearly between liability and being subject to suit was misleading and accounted for physician distrust when the hospital attorney explained the situation.

The subject of medical staff member exposure to suit and liability should be reviewed regularly with the staff. In some states there is an indication that, in addition to judicial recognition of the justification for the protection afforded by peer review statutes, courts are less prone to allow suits alleging malice in peer review to go to trial absent specific and detailed allegations. Thus, a mere statement of malice in the complaint may be insufficient to avoid summary dismissal of a physician's suit.

6.

Most physicians under review will allege anticompetitive behavior and personality differences to explain why they have been singled out. The board and the hospital's attorney should seek assurance that there is merit in the charges against a physician and that the witnesses will be able to withstand competent cross-examination. This is best accomplished by obtaining an outside consultant, board-certified in the specialty, who has no connection with the local medical community. If the consultant confirms the findings of the medical staff, it is very likely that the case against the physician is strong.

In many instances the fact that there is an outside consultant, who will be testifying about the physician's performance, is sufficient to resolve the matter, with the doctor either resigning or accepting appropriate supervision of his exercise of privileges.

7.

Finally, there are some avenues to pursue to solve the apparent Dr. Brown hearing dilemma:

- The hearing could be held under the aegis of the court, with the appointment of a master. Under such a procedure, the hospital surrenders some control.
- The hearing could be conducted by a committee of the board. This creates a problem because of the panel members' lack of knowledge of medicine, but it does take place within the hospital environment and is not an abdication of the institution's responsibility. An objective medical consultant can be provided to assist the committee.
- The board could hire a panel of physicians from outside the medical community to act as the hearing committee.

Given the history of the Dr. Green dispute, the hospital almost certainly should seek to obtain a judicial order to conduct the hearing in accordance with the second or third options so as to minimize subsequent challenge by Dr. Brown in the event of a recommendation and decision adverse to him.

Case 5

The Physician with a Very Special Interest

PERSONAE

Charles Carr, retiring board president of Community Hospital
Larry Coleman, hospital attorney
Jane Davis, medical record librarian
Dr. Martin Lee, surgeon, protagonist
Carl Lewis, attorney for Dr. Lee
Judge Jacob Roth, heard petition for injunction
Fred. St. Clair, secretary, then president, of hospital board
Jack Stackhouse, attorney-consultant for hospital
Harry Taylor, hospital administrator

Harry Taylor, the administrator of Community Hospital, was not particularly keen about calling the secretary of his board, Fred St. Clair, but felt he needed to talk to one of the trustees, both to provide a sounding board for his concern and to obtain guidance. St. Clair was a long-time member of the hospital board and his executive position in a substantial corporation included responsibility for personnel matters. Taylor thought that someone familiar with personnel could be of considerable assistance.

Community was one of three hospitals in a city of 75,000 population. To be frank about it, Community Hospital ranked third and last in reputation and in the quality of its medical staff. It did not enjoy the support of the city's top families and key business leaders. Nevertheless, it made a contribution to the community and an objective observer could say that Taylor administered the hospital in satisfactory fashion. It operated in the black and no scandal, alleged or actual, about its operation had ever been raised.

St. Clair took the call from Taylor. After an exchange of pleasantries, St. Clair, who had received not more than one or two calls a year from Taylor about hospital matters, sought to find out quickly what had prompted this one. Taylor explained briefly that he believed they had a problem with a physician on the medical staff. He said he was picking up stray pieces of information about the conduct of a surgeon named Dr. Martin Lee, who in the past had attracted some attention because of his difficulty in complying with the hospital's rules and procedures.

Taylor said some of the troublesome conduct consisted of nasty behavior toward nurses and other hospital employees both during surgery and on various hospital units where Dr. Lee's patients were assigned. He told St. Clair he had interviewed two nurses who, very reluctantly, had given him the facts of two instances of such behavior. The nurses, he said, had told him that they didn't want to make trouble and were concerned about repercussions that might follow because of their reports of Dr. Lee's conduct.

At this point the board secretary asked Taylor whether it was his opinion that Dr. Lee's conduct was likely to recur or whether these were isolated instances. Taylor responded that if they were only isolated instances, he would not have bothered to call and that he believed the likelihood was strong that there would be more incidents and that the board might have to make a decision either to discipline Dr. Lee or not to reappoint him for the next medical staff year.

The administrator told St. Clair he did not want to prejudge these matters but needed informal guidance as to how to proceed. St. Clair suggested Taylor contact the president of the board, a businessman named Charles Carr, and propose that a meeting of the board's Executive Committee and the administrator be held to consider what steps, if any, should be taken.

* * * * *

The Executive Committee met several days later. The hospital never had had a situation in which a member of the medical staff had been disciplined through board action and there never had been a suspension or revocation of privileges or a denial of reappointment. The Executive Committee members who attended were concerned, if such a step were to be contemplated, that there be firm legal grounds for any such action.

Community Hospital did not have an attorney regularly providing legal services. There was one practicing attorney on the board and, occasionally, hospital legal matters were referred to him. He was not compensated for legal services he provided and he had played only a minor role in hospital affairs. Taylor suggested that an outside attorney familiar with hospital legal matters be consulted to provide guidance to him and the committee as to the hospital's legal position if any action were to be taken against Dr. Lee. The consensus view of the Executive Committee was that Taylor should find such an attorney and report back to the president of the board, who would instruct the administrator as to the next step.

That day Taylor telephoned Jack Stackhouse, an attorney in a nearby state who spoke on medical staff matters at hospital meetings and whom he had once heard. Taylor described the kinds of incidents that had come to his attention and the position of the Executive Committee. The attorney told Taylor it was essential that the hospital's bylaws and the medical staff bylaws, rules, and regulations be reviewed to determine the bases for taking action and procedural steps that would have to be followed if the board moved against Dr. Lee.

Taylor then spoke with Carr, the board president, who proposed that they, St. Clair, and any other members of the Executive Committee who wished to attend, pay a visit to Stackhouse. Carr urged Taylor to be as discreet as possible about the fact that an attorney's assistance was being sought.

Taylor was enthusiastic about the idea of obtaining legal advice and was able to arrange a meeting for the following week at Stackhouse's office. The attorney instructed Taylor to bring copies of a variety of hospital documents.

On the day specified, the meeting was held, attended by Taylor, St. Clair, Carr, and one other board member. Stackhouse did not know anything about Community Hospital and, as the first step in acquainting himself with the situation, asked for and was given a brief oral history of the institution. He learned that Community Hospital had been established shortly after World War II for use by physicians who had limited recognition within the community and who needed more extensive opportunities for hospital practice than they were able to obtain at the two major institutions in the city. Those two hospitals had not discouraged the development of a third one, in part because it gave them an opportunity to restrict their staffs.

The hospital bylaws and medical staff bylaws had been adopted in 1948, when the hospital opened. The medical staff bylaws had been revised once in the late 1950s but not since, although at the present time, in 1964, consideration was being given to adopting a new set or, at a minimum, extensively revising the existing set.

Stackhouse pointed out to his visitors that the only provisions in the hospital bylaws dealing with appointment and other medical staff matters stated that the governing board would appoint physicians based on recommendations from the medical staff. The medical staff bylaws provided in very simple language for recommendations to the board for appointment and reappointment of physicians. The bylaws were silent on revocation or suspension of privileges or of appointment, except that a physician could be removed from the staff for "cause." The bylaws provided no procedures for conducting a disciplinary investigation or reviewing recommendations for discipline.

The result of the meeting was Stackhouse's recommendation that the medical staff bylaws be revised promptly to incorporate more detailed provisions dealing with the appointment and reappointment processes and that sections be added to cover disciplinary action against physicians who violated medical staff and hospital rules or conducted themselves in ways that created risks or dangers to patient care or to the smooth functioning of the institution. The attorney also suggested that, with respect to Dr. Lee, no immediate action be taken but that upon receipt of the recommendation of the medical staff for reappointment or denial of reappointment, the board be prepared to meet to assess this physician's performance and conduct as part of the reappointment process. He advised that Taylor find a way to diplomatically acquaint Dr. Lee with the fact that he now was under some scrutiny and that he should seek to mend his ways.

The meeting broke up with the board members greatly enthusiastic about bringing their medical staff and corporate bylaws up to date. They agreed that these documents had been neglected for years and no longer were suitable for the governance and operation of the hospital, at least for medical staff matters.

* * * * *

There was no further communication between Taylor or anyone else on behalf of Community Hospital and Stackhouse for nearly a year and a half. Then, in the spring of 1966, Taylor telephoned the attorney and told him that the situation involving Dr. Lee had become much more serious. He added that St. Clair, who had advanced from being the board's secretary to becoming its president, had directed him to contact Stackhouse because he felt they needed a lawyer. Stackhouse asked whether any of the hospital documents had been revised since their visit and was told that no action had been taken, although committees of both the board and the medical staff were looking into possible changes in both sets of bylaws. In response to a question, Taylor told Stackhouse that he had talked with Dr. Lee, who had denied any improper conduct, and that the physician had been routinely reappointed to the staff for both 1965 and 1966.

Stackhouse agreed to provide assistance to Community Hospital but on condition that a local attorney be designated to participate in the handling of the Lee case. Taylor said such an arrangement could be made easily although there was no local lawyer that he and board leaders believed to be particularly knowledgeable about hospital medical staff matters. He also expressed the view that for local, political reasons, attorneys from firms represented on the boards of the two other hospitals should not be involved. Stackhouse said that almost any attorney acceptable to Community Hospital would be acceptable to him, and a meeting was scheduled at Taylor's office for the following week at which the administrator would detail the incidents that were creating concern. Taylor said he would try to have a local attorney for the hospital present.

Taylor had a week to prepare for Stackhouse's visit. He was not an administrator of the cool, business school, socially adept genre. Rather, he was a rough-hewn type who had left a modest position in industry to become director of housekeeping services of a hospital. Over the next 10 years he had learned his hospital administration on the job, moving from one institution to another, always to a higher position. When he had been hired by Community four years earlier, he had been selected in part because, although he seemed competent, he was also willing to work at a lower salary and without a number of perquisites demanded by some of the applicants, who were preferred by many on the board. One thing that certainly could be said on behalf of Taylor was that he was very conscientious and thorough.

During the week in which he was to marshal facts for the meeting with Stackhouse, he produced three notebooks containing copies of portions of certain patient records, notes he had made of the comments that had been given at the most recent survey by the Joint Commission on Accreditation of Hospitals, copies of summaries of statements by nursing personnel, copies of the listings of patient charts incomplete more that 15 days that were posted regularly on the first day of each month, and copies of several confidential communications sent to him by the director of nursing. All of these items concerned Dr. Lee and, in Taylor's opinion, supported the view that the surgeon had to be dealt with.

Dr. Lee was in his early 40s. He had ranked very high in his medical school class, completed sufficient graduate training to become eligible for board certification, and had in fact become certified as a general surgeon. While his personal life was not fully known to Taylor and others at the hospital, there were murmurings about his marital situation that suggested it was rocky. According to the rumors, his wife was about to seek a divorce and it was fairly well known that he had made social or sexual overtures to a number of female hospital employees during the preceding year or two. Dr. Lee was not considered popular with his physician colleagues; rather, he was a loner who did not appear to have any close friends within the hospital community.

Taylor's quest for an attorney did not meet with initial success. He talked with the president, St. Clair, the past president, Carr, and several other board members. They did not know particularly what they were looking for, recognizing that the lawyers who represented the two other institutions in town were the only ones who evidently had any experience with hospital affairs. They also were fairly confident that Stackhouse would be able to play a large role in the events that would be likely to take place. As a result, their thinking at the time was that an attorney with some administrative law experience should be found to handle the situation even if he were not to serve as the hospital's regular lawyer in the future. The opinion of the one attorney on the board was not solicited at all, apparently because during his tenure on the board he had not demonstrated much interest in the hospital.

Larry Coleman was a successful local attorney who represented utility companies and other clients that from time to time were involved with the state bureaucracy. He was regarded as patient and thorough. Coleman was approached by Taylor and after a brief discussion agreed to attend the meeting with Stackhouse. He did not commit himself to anything more, saying that unless he felt that he could give the hospital the type of representation and counsel it needed, he would have to withdraw. Taylor delivered to Coleman a package consisting of copies of the hospital and medical staff bylaws, the state hospital licensing regulations, the then current set of Joint Commission standards, and various other materials that he told the attorney would be worth looking at in preparation for the meeting. He did not send copies of the notebooks containing the items relating to Dr. Lee's activities.

Up to this point there had been no contact between Taylor and any members of the hospital's medical staff regarding the procedure that might be followed in dealing with Dr. Lee. Taylor had discussed with St. Clair whether to involve the chief of staff. St. Clair had said, "Until we know where we stand legally, there is no reason to get the doctors all upset." Since Taylor did not have a particularly high opinion of the current chief of staff and knew that, as a general practitioner, he referred a considerable number of cases to Dr. Lee, he went along with the board president's position.

The day before the meeting was to be held, Taylor, in order to maintain secrecy—which at that point was quite strict—called Stackhouse and suggested that the session be held at Coleman's office rather than at the hospital.

* * * * *

The following day Stackhouse, Taylor, and Coleman met at the attorney's office. After an exchange of greetings Taylor opened a box that contained the three notebooks filled with the items he had collected that related in one way or another to Dr. Lee. This collection soon became known as the "Lee file."

The notes on the Joint Commission survey indicated that the surveyor had specifically mentioned that Dr. Lee had a poorer record than any other member of the medical staff with regard to completing his medical records within 15 days after discharge. This was a standard based upon state hospital licensing agency regulations. Because of this chart completion failing, the surveyor had asked to see several of Dr. Lee's charts. After brief examination, the surveyor had told Taylor that, in his opinion, even the so-called completed ones were incomplete as a practical matter because of their sketchiness. In addition, he pointed out that in several instances ordinary preoperative diagnostic procedures were not evidenced on the chart. He also noted that the relatively substantial incidence of removal of what laboratory studies indicated were nonpathological tissues suggested that Dr. Lee was at best careless in deciding when to operate. While he did not put anything about Dr. Lee's surgery in his actual report, the surveyor told Taylor that he should get the surgeon to "shape up'' because he was the kind who, unless kept under a tight rein, would go from poor to bad.

Subsequent to the survey, the lists of medical records incomplete more than 15 days indicated that in most months Dr. Lee continued to have more such tardy charts than anyone else on the staff. Although his performance in completing medical records had improved somewhat during the most recent four or five months, he still appeared regularly, and prominently, at or near the top of the delinquent list.

The notes from the conversations with members of the nursing staff indicated that many young female patients who had their tonsils and adenoids removed by Dr. Lee complained of pain in the area of their vaginas after they had returned to the units. This could not be readily explained, given the nature of the procedure being performed. When nurses brought this discomfort to Dr. Lee's attention, he had told them not to worry about it and that he would explain ''everything'' to the parents. However, the nurses had told Taylor that a number of parents also had inquired of them about their daughters' complaints and had expressed concern. Incidents of this type had been occurring for more than a year.

Other notes based on conversations with nurses described incidents where Dr. Lee had used foul language in the operating room in chastising them for alleged failure to carry out his orders properly and indicated that he had treated other OR personnel similarly. One of Taylor's notes indicated that Dr. Lee had struck a technician immediately after a procedure, according to the operating room supervisor, but the technician denied she had been touched. She told the administrator only that Dr. Lee was obnoxious and if at all possible she did not want to work on any cases with him again.

The ''Lee file'' also contained notes of conversations with nurses who reported that older women also had complained occasionally of discomfort or odd feeling in the vaginal area after abdominal or gynecological surgery. Taylor's extracts from selected patient records revealed that for practically every adult female patient upon whom Dr. Lee had performed surgery, the operating report had a standard entry, ''adhesions were released around clitoris.'' Nothing in the history or physical examination report for any of these patients indicated a clinical reason for this procedure.

Patient records also revealed that Dr. Lee had performed a great many of the female sterilization procedures done at the hospital. The consent forms that patients had signed often did not mention specifically that sterility—loss of the ability to procreate—would result. The procedures were entered on the form solely in medical terminology.

The file memoranda from the director of nursing dealt with three subjects:

1. The releasing of clitoral adhesions and the nurses' concern about the frequency about which this procedure was performed on older women patients
2. The incidents involving vaginal area discomfort described to nurses by young female patients
3. Complaints by nurses about conversations with, and physical touching by, Dr. Lee, mostly in and near the operating room.

The nurses said he often suggested that one of them join him for dinner or spend an evening with him. A number of nurses who reported such overtures were married and they, particularly, felt that these were serious invitations rather than casual, jocular propositions. Some also had mentioned to the director of nursing that Dr. Lee would pat them on the back or shoulder and occasionally pinch them in a not all together playful manner. The nurses who had complained said they were only seeking to have Dr. Lee "lay off" and didn't want to make a "big deal" over these incidents.

Taylor had Stackhouse and Coleman review the contents of the notebooks carefully and answered questions that they raised as they read the materials. He then asked the attorneys what they thought. Coleman, the first to respond, said "They could hang his ass" for what he was doing and expressed shock that Dr. Lee's behavior had been tolerated for so long. Stackhouse, more conservative in his response, said he thought there were two questions: (1)Were there grounds that would bring Community Hospital to take action against Dr. Lee? (2) If Community wanted to get rid of Dr. Lee, was the law sufficiently on the hospital's side so that it would be successful?

Stackhouse then asked, "What does this business about releasing adhesions around the clitoris mean?"

"I've looked into it," Taylor answered. "The purpose is to free the clitoris so that the woman will receive greater clitoral stimulation during intercourse and, presumably, more sexual satisfaction. It is evidently legitimate activity for a physician."

"For 8 and 9 year-old girls too?" Stackhouse inquired.

"That's a question that bothers me, too," Taylor replied

Stackhouse then reviewed, primarily for Coleman's benefit, the developing medical staff law. He pointed out that courts in New Jersey were recognizing due process rights for physicians. He felt that the evidence that Taylor had compiled would certainly support a determination adverse to Dr. Lee. He said that if action were to be instituted, it would be advisable to establish a set of procedures for holding a hearing and for a board decision-making course so the hospital would not be subject to challenge on a due process argument.

The attorney pointed out that the state in which Community Hospital was located had not had any reported decisions up to that time involving staff disciplinary or appointment or reappointment controversies. He was concerned for the hospital's possibility of success in dealing with Dr. Lee and, if there were to be a higher court decision in the event the surgeon challenged Community's action, that the state courts be generally supportive of the concept of hospital responsibility for monitoring and controlling members of the medical staff.

Coleman asked Stackhouse to provide him with legal references. He told Taylor he was very interested in being involved in any proceeding regarding Dr. Lee's conduct. He said that while he was a novice in the medical area, he believed he not only would be serving as an attorney for the hospital but also would be contributing to the community by helping to rid it of a "rogue" physician.

A brief discussion of what was to take place next followed. Taylor said the hospital board would have to decide whether to move against Dr. Lee and, until that decision was made, he saw no reason for doing anything further, except that Coleman should familiarize himself in detail with the notebook materials, the hospital's documents, and relevant law. Stackhouse agreed to provide Coleman with references and other materials.

Taylor, on the way to his car after the meeting, asked Stackhouse when his flight was leaving. Stackhouse said he had about two hours. Taylor told him a special dinner meeting of the board's Executive Committee was scheduled that night to review the Lee situation. The administrator said St. Clair, the board president, wanted Stackhouse to attend and that the attorney should shift his flight to the next day, if at all possible, so he could be present. Stackhouse inquired why Coleman was not to attend. Taylor replied that, because it had not been known whether Coleman would be willing to serve as attorney, it had been decided that Stackhouse alone be the counselor at this special session.

* * * * *

That evening, five of the six members of the board's Executive Committee, plus Taylor and Stackhouse, met for drinks and dinner in a private room at the hotel. Taylor reviewed the notebook materials he had provided to Stackhouse and Coleman. He said it would be up to the board members to determine whether some action should be taken against Dr. Lee and, if so, what that action should be. St. Clair, whose idea it had been to have the meeting with Stackhouse present, asked the attorney to review the hospital's legal situation in these circumstances.

Stackhouse did so, the gist of his remarks being that, in his opinion, there were ample grounds for action to remove Dr. Lee from the staff and that, if proper procedures were followed, there was little doubt that the hospital would prevail in court if the surgeon were to contest such an action. Several board members asked questions of Stackhouse, focusing on their concern about the effect on the hospital of the public's becoming aware of Dr. Lee's activities if action were taken against the surgeon and if he were to take the case to court. Stackhouse several times mentioned that Dr. Lee had a lot at stake, too, if the matter were exposed to the public.

While no formal votes were taken, it appeared that, after discussion, a clear majority of the board members present—led by Carr, the past president—favored taking disciplinary action against Dr. Lee. As the consensus formed, Stackhouse thought the meeting was nearly over and that he could retire for the night.

At this point Carr asked St. Clair, almost as an aside, whether he thought that public airing of the Lee problem would affect the hospital's planned drive to raise funds to construct additional facilities. St. Clair indicated that this was a matter that deserved attention and for nearly an hour the board members expressed their views as to whether the proposed expansion would be jeopardized.

Gradually, the consensus moved toward giving Dr. Lee one more chance. It was suggested that several board members meet with him privately to point out that his failings and improper behavior were known to them and that his actions no longer would be tolerated.

Stackhouse was thoroughly worn out, particularly because of the indecisiveness of the Executive Committee. He had remained silent during the discussion about the Lee problem and the hospital's expansion but finally could contain himself no longer.

He said there was little reason to believe that Dr. Lee would improve without something more decisive than a warning conversation. The key member of the board in most of the discussion had been Carr, who earlier had supported action against the surgeon and then had raised the subject of the expansion. It appeared he had moved toward seeking to avoid an open confrontation. At this point Carr said he thought a formal vote should be taken on Dr. Lee. He said Taylor now, in a sense, was out on a limb with Dr. Lee and that although secrecy had been maintained fairly well, an increasing number of persons in the hospital family were aware of the fact that the board was considering the situation.

St. Clair was reluctant to put any question to vote but, at Carr's urging, said he would do so if that was the will of the board members. At this point Carr made a motion to direct Taylor to prepare charges against Dr. Lee on behalf of the board so it could revoke the surgeon's appointment. Stackhouse's opinion was not sought at all at this point. The motion was seconded and St. Clair asked whether there was need for further discussion. No one replied. St. Clair asked for a show of hands. At first, only Carr raised his hand. Then another board member did so, and over the next 30 seconds all the others, one by one, raised their hands. St. Clair then said he was in accord with the rest of the members of the Executive Committee and, after a round of self-congratulations, the meeting adjourned.

Taylor took Stackhouse aside and asked whether he would be willing to provide further assistance to Coleman and himself so that everything would go well. Stackhouse agreed to do so but indicated he felt the board was rather insecure about its action, irresolute, and likely to act like a pendulum on the subject of how to deal with Dr. Lee. He told Taylor there were many details to take care of and that he felt confident he could work with Coleman.

* * * * *

During the following two weeks Stackhouse and Coleman held several telephone conversations to decide upon the specific charges that would be brought against Dr. Lee. They listed a considerable number:

- the lack of evidence that informed consent had been obtained for sterilization procedures, at least as far as the consent form used by Dr. Lee was concerned
- the failure to obtain consent for the release of clitoral adhesions for older female patients
- the performance of some type of procedure around the clitoris of young female patients without obtaining consent from the parents
- the failure to enter on the charts of young female patients, either in the operating room report or in the discharge summary, that some procedure had been performed around the clitoris
- the absence of evidence in the charts of medical need for the sterilization procedures on many of the women
- the absence in the charts of evidence of medical need to perform any procedure in the clitoral area on the young female patients
- the failure to complete records within 15 days after discharge
- four specific instances of physical touching of, and conversational advances to, members of the nursing staff.

Drafts of specifications for these charges were prepared by Coleman with the assistance of Stackhouse. For each specification, references to particular patient charts, the names of nursing personnel, and references to the state hospital licensing regulations describing what constituted a proper chart for hospitalized patients were set forth, to indicate the sources of evidence. For some of these instances, it appeared advisable, if not essential, to obtain physicians who would testify in an expert sense to support the charges. This was particularly true on the sterilization procedures and the nature and extent of the information to be provided patients, or their legal representatives, before effective consent would be present.

It also was considered advisable to have a physician testify in some detail about the procedures around the clitoris, specifically because of the connotations such activity would have for the board members.

Coleman delivered a draft of the specifications to Taylor at his office. They discussed them at length and the administrator raised a number of objections. He said he had conducted further informal interviews with the nurses and that none of them were willing to testify at any proceeding on Dr. Lee's activities or overtures. They said they felt this would be embarrassing to them and that they were seriously concerned about possible retaliation, not only by Dr. Lee but also by other staff members who they felt would not hesitate (1) to make unfounded complaints about their professional performance and (2) to stimulate controversy concerning them. Taylor said he was unable to convince the nurses that he and the board would stand behind them completely if physicians sought to make difficulties for them.

As to some of the other specifications, Taylor said he could not be certain that any members of the medical staff would be willing to testify as friendly witnesses for the hospital against Dr. Lee. Coleman saw at this point that much of the case was going to fall apart even before any hearing was held. He suggested that Taylor call Stackhouse and they conducted a three-way conversation by phone. After Taylor reported his difficulties, Stackhouse suggested that the charges be limited to those that clearly were violations of either a hospital rule or the state hospital licensing agency regulations and that no further attempts be made to obtain witnesses to testify about medical practices or specific events involving the nurses.

From this conversation emerged a much shorter list of charges:

- Dr. Lee had not maintained proper medical records in that the patients' histories, reports of physical examinations, and provisional diagnoses showed no reason for the procedures. This would group cases where sterilizations were performed without any indications in the chart, and where adhesions were released for older women patients.
- Dr. Lee had not maintained proper medical records in that procedures were performed and not recorded in the charts at all, either in the operative report or discharge summary.
- Dr. Lee's records remained incomplete more than 15 days as shown on the lists of incomplete charts posted monthly. This was to be supported by a list of charts, by number, indicating for each when the 15-day period had ended and the length of time after that during which the record remained incomplete. This supporting list covered a year and contained 160 chart numbers.

The subject of charges based upon possibly not obtaining proper consent for the sterilization procedures was discussed at considerable length. Stackhouse expressed the concern that such charges would require participation by patients and that this in turn might lead to their bringing lawsuits against the hospital, as well as against Dr. Lee, because Community permitted him to perform sterilization procedures without consent. Coleman and Stackhouse agreed that some of the female patients who had been sterilized not only might not have had any medical indications for the procedure but also might well not have known beforehand that they would be sterilized, or still were not aware that they had been. In their opinion, the liability risks militated against pursuing consent aspects of the sterilization cases.

Coleman agreed to put the specifications in final form and Taylor said he then would talk with St. Clair about a date for a hearing far enough in the future so that Dr. Lee would not be able to claim that he had had no opportunity to prepare his case. Stackhouse then asked a series of questions that he said needed prompt answers. Among them were: How were the charges to be given to Dr. Lee? Who would serve as prosecutor on behalf of the hospital by presenting the evidence to support the charges against Dr. Lee? Who would constitute the hearing body? Various other questions involved procedural matters.

Taylor's opinion was that there was no way to draw a hearing panel from among members of the medical staff. Even though Dr. Lee was not very popular, he was someone whom most members of the medical staff clearly did not want to cross in any way. The administrator was instructed to inquire of St. Clair whether a committee drawn from the board should serve as the hearing panel or whether the entire board would serve.

Coleman suggested that the procedures generally followed in state administrative matters be adhered to in the proceeding and that the hospital arrange for a court reporter and furnish the room much like a courtroom. He recommended that the rules of evidence for state administrative proceedings be followed. He also proposed that he present the case on behalf of the hospital by introducing charts and other evidence, conducting the examination of any hospital witnesses, and cross-examining those on behalf of Dr. Lee, if any testified.

Taylor inquired about Stackhouse's role in the proceedings. Coleman said he believed he could handle the hearing completely by himself and that he thought the presence of Stackhouse as an outsider from another state, might raise difficulties for some members of the hospital board in that it might give them an excuse to be less strict with Dr. Lee than they might be otherwise. The administrator, who was inclined to have Stackhouse participate actively in the proceeding, decided not to pursue the matter further. Stackhouse said he was perfectly willing to drop out of the picture at any time, particularly as far as the hearing was concerned. The subject of his participation was then dropped.

The next day Taylor, not fully confident in Coleman's ability to go it alone at this point, called Stackhouse and said he wanted the attorney to be present the day of the hearing. Stackhouse agreed to do so. The administrator said he wanted Stackhouse involved to the extent of reviewing with Coleman the final plans for presentation of evidence and to be available at the hearing location, although he could remain in the background. Stackhouse said he would not accept such an involvement unless Coleman agreed. The conversation ended with Taylor saying he would speak to Coleman and that one of them would call him. The next day Coleman telephoned Stackhouse and said he appreciated any assistance Stackhouse could give on the day of the hearing.

* * * * *

Plans moved ahead for the hearing. St. Clair chose a date three weeks in the future, on a day when it was likely a good number of the board could be present. The notion of selecting a committee of three or five to hear the case and to make a recommendation to the board was rejected quickly in favor of having as many board members present as possible. The rationale for this was the belief by St. Clair and Carr that all the board members would want to be able to make their own decisions based on the evidence, and not be influenced by a "select few" who would participate in the hearing if a panel were to be selected.

Coleman advised Taylor that, instead of mailing or in some other fashion delivering the charges to Dr. Lee at his office or home, the surgeon be invited to Taylor's office and, in the presence of the administrator's secretary, be given an envelope containing the charges and notification of the date, time, and location of the hearing. Taylor was very reluctant to do so, but finally agreed.

With the final set of charges drawn, the plans for the hearing well along, and the date having been selected, Taylor invited Dr. Lee to see him early on a Thursday morning. When the surgeon arrived, Taylor handed him an envelope containing the charges and the notice of the hearing. The notice stated that the hearing would be held at the hospital, exactly 21 days from the date on which Dr. Lee received the charges, at 7 P.M. The notice also said Dr. Lee could be represented by counsel if he so desired.

As Dr. Lee opened the envelope and read the charges, he looked up at Taylor from time to time with a grin on his face. Finally, after he finished reading, he said to the administrator:

"From now on it's all downhill for you. You'll be out of this hospital in six months and we'll make sure you will never get a job in this part of the state again. You are such a dumb bastard you don't know anything about medical practice."

At that point Dr. Lee stormed out of Taylor's office.

Taylor immediately called Coleman and told him of Dr. Lee's initial response to the charges. Coleman said the surgeon probably would take a day or so to digest what was going on and then find an attorney to assist him. He also told Taylor that it would be advisable to keep out of Dr. Lee's way, although he should not ignore violations of the hospital's rules and policies by the surgeon.

Taylor then called Stackhouse who, after hearing of the session, said the administrator should not have expected a very different response and should not be concerned. To Taylor, Stackhouse seemed mildly disturbed about the way the charges and notice were delivered to Dr. Lee, but there was no explicit criticism of Coleman's advice.

The following Monday, Taylor received a telephone call from a local attorney named Carl Lewis, who told him he had become counsel to Dr. Lee and wanted to know who was counsel for the hospital because it was necessary for him to prepare for the hearing. Taylor referred Lewis to Coleman and then immediately called both St. Clair and Coleman to let them know that Dr. Lee was now represented by counsel. Coleman told Taylor that from that time on he should not say anything to Lewis and should refer all inquiries or questions about Dr. Lee or the hearing to him.

Lewis was a former assistant district attorney who had won the Democratic nomination for district attorney in the previous primary but had lost in the general election, although he had fared well considering the county was overwhelmingly Republican. He was well known for an active and financially rewarding criminal practice. He did not limit his work to the immediate locality but handled cases all over the state and occasionally was involved in major cases in other states as well.

During his call to Coleman, Lewis attempted to work out a settlement. He said Dr. Lee would agree to forego any practices that the hospital felt were improper although he would not admit that anything he had done in the past was incorrect. Lewis said that as far as Dr. Lee was concerned these were trivial matters and he was willing to bring an end to the controversy by making such an agreement. Coleman said he would discuss the proposal with the hospital and, after the conversation was concluded, called Taylor. Recalling the indecision of the board's Executive Committee at the meeting at which it was finally determined to move against Dr. Lee, Taylor said he felt the proposal would have to be rejected and that he preferred not to bring it to the board's attention.

Coleman responded that Taylor was only the administrator and that, since the board had decided to bring charges through its Executive Committee, he had no choice but to discuss the offer with St. Clair at least.

A meeting was promptly held at which St. Clair, Carr, Taylor, and Coleman were present. Lewis's proposal was discussed and the current and past board presidents agreed that the matter had gone too far for the hospital to drop the charges in return for Dr. Lee's agreement "to go and sin no more," as St.

Clair put it, particularly since the surgeon was not even willing to admit that he had erred in the past. The hospital's response was communicated to Lewis and the stage was set for the hearing.

Stackhouse arrived in town at noon on the day of the hearing and immediately went to Coleman's office. They discussed procedural details. Stackhouse agreed he would not participate in the session in any way, he would not be introduced to anyone, and would sit unobtrusively in the rear of the room only to observe.

Stackhouse then asked who would preside. When Coleman answered "St. Clair," Stackhouse inquired how "this layman" would know how to rule on evidentiary issues and procedural matters. Coleman was surprised by the question; he apparently had not given any thought to it before. He suggested that the attorney member of the board be asked to preside, and Stackhouse agreed this might be a solution. Coleman telephoned St. Clair, who rejected the idea of anyone else but him presiding. He told Coleman that "common sense will be sufficient. We don't want to make this too legal." Coleman practically pleaded with the board president to have the attorney preside, but St. Clair was adamant. Except for this subject, Coleman and Stackhouse were basically satisfied that the procedural preparations for the hearing were satisfactory.

* * * * *

The board members began to arrive at the hospital meeting room where the hearing was to take place shortly before 7 P.M. They all were introduced to Coleman by Taylor and were seated at a long table at one side of the room. Two counsel tables had been set up and a witness chair provided. A court reporter hired by the hospital also was present to make a complete record of the hearing.

At exactly 7 o'clock, Lewis and Dr. Lee entered the room, followed immediately by nine members of the medical staff of Community Hospital. After time for introducing everyone to everyone else, except Stackhouse, St. Clair convened the hearing at 7:15 P.M. A few other persons also entered during the introductions.

St. Clair began by reading the charges. He then asked both Coleman and Lewis whether they wished to make opening statements. Before Coleman could respond, Lewis rose and said Dr. Lee was appearing under protest. He pointed to the absence of any hearing or appeal provisions in the medical staff bylaws and said the ad hoc procedures established were not adequate to provide his client with due process. He then introduced a court reporter he had brought with him and demanded that she make the only record of the hearing. After a brief argument between Lewis and Coleman, St. Clair ruled that both reporters would be allowed to make their records.

Coleman made a brief opening statement indicating the evidence he would introduce regarding the three charges against Dr. Lee. Lewis followed with an opening statement in which he said his client was a highly regarded member of the medical profession and that a substantial number of members of the medical staff of Community Hospital were prepared to testify on his behalf. Lewis charged that Taylor and some members of the medical staff, whom he preferred not to identify, were participating in a conspiracy to "get" Dr. Lee and that for the hospital board to be used to settle a private vendetta directed against the surgeon was a disservice to the community.

"When the public learns of the plot against Dr. Lee, as they certainly will, the reputation of Community Hospital will be forever tarnished," he said. "Small men are going to destroy this fine institution."

It was evident to Stackhouse at the rear of the room that at least some of the board members were very troubled by Lewis's remarks.

When Lewis finished, St. Clair directed Coleman to begin presentation of evidence. Coleman read the charges, then asked Lewis to agree to entering in the record as evidence certain provisions of the state hospital licensing regulations. Excerpts from the provisions offered were as follows:

1. A complete medical record shall be compiled for each patient admitted as an inpatient. The medical record shall contain the following:

   Complaint
   Present and past history
   Report of physical examination
   Provisional diagnosis
   Medical treatment
   Complete record of surgery
   Progress notes
   Nurses' notes
   Final diagnosis

2. Medical records must be completed no more than 15 days after discharge.

Lewis agreed to admission of the material but only after lengthy remarks to the effect that the state hospital licensing agency could not interfere with the practice of medicine by a licensed physician and that the regulations applied only to hospitals, not to physicians.

Coleman reread the first charge, that Dr. Lee had failed to maintain proper medical records in that the patients' histories, reports of physical examinations, and provisional diagnoses showed no reason for the procedures. He called as witness Jane Davis, the hospital medical record librarian. She had prepared extracts from the records of a number of patients who had been sterilized, for whom there were no entries indicating any medical need for the procedure, as well as extracts from several additional records in which Dr. Lee had made entries that adhesions were released around the clitoris but where there were no entries indicating the need for such procedures.

Ms. Davis described the process by which the material was extracted from the records and the system used for preparing the extracts. Coleman moved to introduce the extracts into evidence and Lewis raised no objection. When Coleman asked the medical record librarian what constituted indications for the procedures, specifically the sterilizations, Lewis objected. After a lengthy argument Lewis agreed to her testimony, but only with respect to what usually was present in the records of women patients of other physicians on the medical staff who performed sterilizations. He was able to gain St. Clair's agreement to instruct the board that only the absence of entries in the records, not whether there actually were indications for the procedures on the patients, could be established by the librarian's testimony.

Coleman then introduced extracts from the records of several young female patients, without objection by Lewis, as relevant to the charge of failure to maintain proper medical records in that procedures were performed and not noted in the records at all. These patients had received tonsillectomies and adenoidectomies yet their operative report and discharge summary contained no mention of any procedure performed in the clitoral area and for which there were nursing notes indicating discomfort in that area. Ms. Davis testified that she had selected only T and A patients' records for which there were nursing notes about clitoral area discomfort. Coleman then introduced into evidence lists of records by physician name, incomplete for more than 15 days, that were prepared routinely by the librarian. These showed Dr. Lee to have had many incomplete records on almost all of the lists. Coleman then said he was finished with the witness.

Lewis and Dr. Lee had appeared rather bored by the presentation of evidence. Before giving Lewis an opportunity to cross-examine the witness, St. Clair asked whether any members of the board had any questions. One board member asked the medical record librarian, "What are clitoral adhesions?"

Before she could answer, Lewis objected on the ground that a medical record librarian was not a physician and therefore was not familiar with medical procedures. St. Clair was somewhat puzzled by Lewis's objection and he looked to Coleman, who rose and said that Ms. Davis should be given the opportunity to answer the question because she was familiar with medical terminology based on her education and experience as a medical record librarian at Community Hospital for several years and at other institutions before that.

St. Clair still was puzzled and didn't seem to know where to turn for guidance. He looked toward the back of the room where Stackhouse was sitting. Stackhouse slowly nodded his head up and down. It was not evident that anyone noticed this exchange. St. Clair then ruled that the Ms. Davis could answer, although the board was to recognize that she was not a medical practitioner. Lewis pursued the objection further, and made a lengthy statement about the "illegality" of lay persons judging the quality of professional medical performance, particularly when they were relying on the testimony of "mere clerks."

Eventually the medical record librarian was given the opportunity to answer the question, which she did by saying, "I don't really know." Lewis and Dr. Lee laughed and Coleman was discomfited.

Lewis began his cross-examination by asking whether charges had been brought against any of the other physicians whose names appeared on the lists of those who had records incomplete more than 15 days. Ms. Davis answered that, as far as she knew, this was the first time formal disciplinary action had been taken against any physician because of incomplete records.

Lewis then turned to the issue of qualifications of the witness to determine whether, from the history, report of physical examination, and other entries, there were indications that sterilization should be performed. Ms. Davis admitted that this was not a subject that was covered in her formal education as a medical record librarian, but said that her familiarity with the records of patients of other physicians who performed the procedures indicated that certain findings or indications usually were present on the chart when there was a sterilization.

Lewis pursued this line of questioning at some length, then turned to the issue of the records that had no indications of any procedures performed in the area of the clitoris or vagina but for which there were nurses' notes indicating discomfort. He repeatedly asked how the nurses, or anyone, could know that procedures had been performed in the area of the clitoris during the patient's time in the operating room if there were no entries in the record. The medical record librarian admitted that this was at best a guess, since in the records themselves—which was all she had reviewed—there were no entries that anything had taken place in the operating room involving that area of the patients' bodies. The board members appeared impressed with Lewis's cross-examination on this issue.

When Lewis finished, Coleman asked whether the records of the younger female patients revealed any entries of complaints or discomfort in the clitoral area before the surgery. The medical record librarian testified that none of the records had such notations.

* * * * *

St. Clair said that if Coleman had no other witnesses or evidence to introduce at that time, it now was Lewis's turn. Lewis reviewed the evidence he would present and its relevance to the charges. First, he said, Dr. Lee was a physician of impeccable professional standards and, second, any procedures he performed in the area of the clitoris were legitimate medical activity. Both, he said, would be established by the testimony of members of the Community Hospital medical staff. He then gestured to the physicians present and said to the board members, "Many of you are their patients and you certainly know how well they can be trusted."

At this point, somewhat carried away by his rhetoric, Lewis said, "There has been innuendo and the raising of suspicion about sexual perversion on the part of Dr. Lee in this proceeding."

Coleman jumped to his feet immediately and said, "I want the record to show clearly, and the board to understand, that the first mention of sexual perversion came from the lips of Dr. Lee's own counsel, and that no remarks of hospital counsel, or testimony, had touched on perversion, and that the word has not been previously used."

Lewis, red in the face at this point, looked over at Dr. Lee, who showed disgust.

Evidently deciding that he said enough, Lewis began to introduce his evidence. Over the course of an hour and a half he had each of the nine members of the medical staff present testify as to their evaluation of Dr. Lee as a physician. They said, in almost identical language, that they considered him to be a very competent physician who performed according to the highest standards of the medical profession. They said that procedures for the release of adhesions around the clitoris were recognized medical practice and that they had been instructed in the techniques in medical school.

On cross-examination each responded, when asked whether it was appropriate that such a procedure be performed on older females without any specific indications, that this was such a minor procedure that no specific indications were required and that entries in records that it had been performed were not even necessary. Lewis objected to questions by Coleman about such procedures on the younger female patients and St. Clair granted the objection.

On the issue of the indications for sterilization, the physicians solidly maintained that, in the absence of having the entire medical record available, they could not make any judgment as to the need for that procedure for the patients whose record extracts had been admitted into evidence. They all maintained, though, that when other procedures were being performed, it was beneficial for the patient, and convenient for the surgeon, to perform the sterilization at that time, rather than to require a separate procedure at a later date.

After these physicians testified, Lewis said he would call Dr. Lee to the stand, but before doing so asked permission to make a short statement and was granted the opportunity by St. Clair. Lewis stated:

"All the evidence in this case is based on records, on pieces of paper. Therefore, the board has before it a bookkeeping rap. The board is well advised to drop the proceeding right at this point, even before Dr. Lee testifies."

Coleman objected, saying that arguments of that sort should be reserved for after all evidence had been introduced. St. Clair agreed and told Lewis to get on with his presentation.

Dr. Lee was then called as a witness.

After Dr. Lee described his medical education, graduate training, and current professional practice, Lewis asked him to explain the procedure for removing adhesions from the clitoral area and the purpose for doing so. Dr. Lee, who had on his lap a large thin package covered with brown wrapping paper, opened it and produced a 4' by 4' medical illustration in color that evoked murmurs from many of those present. Dr. Lee held the illustration so the board members could see it and then began his response.

"Because I recognize that many of you would not or could not know without the assistance of a qualified physician about the procedure for releasing clitoral adhesions, I had this illustration prepared," Dr. Lee said. "It shows the clitoris and surrounding body tissue. As you all know, the clitoris, when stimulated, provides for the female's satisfaction during intercourse and unless it is sufficiently stimulated she cannot achieve orgasm."

Dr. Lee then described in detail the anatomy shown in the illustration for a very attentive board. He had left his chair by this time and was holding the illustration in one hand and pointing as he gave his rather elaborate presentation. Then he returned to the chair and said:

"I have learned as a physician that a source of many problems of women patients is their dissatisfaction with their sexual lives. I recognize this particularly in older women patients who need gynecological procedures, and I have encountered great concern among women patients who are undergoing hysterectomies because they believe they will be less womanly after losing the ability to bear children. This, in turn, has an effect on their sexual lives, which accounts for depression and various other mental conditions."

"Therefore, it is my practice, when performing gynecological and other surgery on women for whom I feel this is a concern, to release adhesions of the clitoris to the surrounding tissue in order that they will have enhanced sexual satisfaction. I also release adhesions occasionally on younger female patients, but only those who are entering puberty. I am making it possible for them, when they become more mature, to avoid impediments to the enjoyment of sexual relations.

"This procedure is clearly within appropriate medical practice and I recall being instructed about it while I was a medical student. If any of you feel that women should be deprived of the opportunity to enjoy sex as much as men, then I may have offended you. However, my duty is to my patients, and their welfare is all that I am concerned with."

When Dr. Lee finished, Lewis asked him to address the three specific charges against him. With regard to the allegation that he had failed to show by entries in the patients' charts that there were reasons for sterilization procedures and release of adhesions around the clitoris, Dr. Lee stated that there certainly were reasons for doing the procedures in all instances and, while the charts might not have been complete in an ideal sense, the procedures always were necessary and were performed in a competent and thorough manner.

The surgeon declared that none of the patients from whose records extracts had been made had complained to him about his professional performance and that, as far as he knew, no complaints have been made to Taylor or to any other person in the hospital administration. He concluded his response to the first charge by saying that physicians take the responsibility for the procedures they perform and that as long as these are done satisfactorily, it is not the business of lay persons to second-guess medical decisions.

Responding to the second charge, the alleged failure to record procedures in the region of the clitoris on younger female patients, Dr. Lee said he did not recall that he had done the procedure for any of the patients from whose records extracts had been made and that, since there was nothing in the charts to indicate that there had been the release of the clitoral adhesions, the charge was completely unfounded. He said that when he released clitoral adhesions on younger female patients, he always made the same entry for the procedure as he did on the records of older female patients.

Lewis then asked Dr. Lee to address the charge that he had failed to complete many records within 15 days after discharge. The surgeon replied that all his records were completed eventually, and that he believed the 15-day requirement was a "technical, impractical rule created not by physicians, but by laymen, who thought that paper work, rather than professional performance, was the key element in medical practice."

He said he felt sorry that so many persons were accepting the notion that requirements such as the completion of records should be imposed on physicians since they interfered with the effective practice of medicine. He said it was his practice, because of the pressure to serve his patients promptly, to allow the records to pile up for a while and then take part of a day off to complete them in large batches. He expressed the opinion that his charts already were complete except for a discharge summary and that the basic information about the patients and their treatments was included.

The board seemed very taken by the strength of Dr. Lee's convictions and his emphasis on putting patient care first. During cross-examination, however, Coleman got the surgeon to admit that entries that would provide an indication for procedures performed were not made, but Dr. Lee was steadfast in asserting that this was strictly a question of how much information needed to be put into the records. He denied performing the release of clitoral adhesions on younger female patients. Coleman questioned him hardly at all about his records being incomplete more than 15 days after discharge.

After Coleman finished his cross-examination St. Clair asked the board members whether any of them had any questions. Two were asked: (1) concerning the method used to release clitoral adhesions and (2) whether there were any risks or dangers to the women. Dr. Lee responded in considerable detail and said the procedure was "risk free."

The board president then asked Coleman and Lewis whether they wanted to make any final remarks for the record. A brief discussion ensued as to who would get the opportunity to speak last and St. Clair ruled that Lewis could have the final word.

In his remarks, Coleman sought to emphasize that the state hospital licensing regulations on completion of records and the nature of the information they should contain, bound both the hospitals and the physicians who were members of the medical staff. The question, he said, was whether Dr. Lee had violated these rules and he said the answer was clear, even from the surgeon's own testimony, that the violations had taken place.

When it was Lewis's turn he played on two themes: (1) that lay persons should not be judging the performance of physicians; only physicians were qualified to judge; (2) the charges were "bookkeeping raps" and it was abusive for a physician to have to appear before the board, hire counsel, and be diverted from regular practice activity because of such minor matters. Lewis said he expected the board to take into consideration the excellent reputation that Dr. Lee enjoyed among his peers as a physician and to decline to impose any disciplinary measures.

The hearing ended with the board, the members of the medical staff, and others in attendance, milling around for several minutes. Stackhouse, who had remained in the rear of the room during the entire proceeding, went into the hall. As Dr. Lee and Lewis were leaving, the surgeon approached Stackhouse and said, "I guess you are the only person I don't know and haven't met." Stackhouse nodded and the two shook hands. Stackhouse did not identify himself and Dr. Lee did not seem to notice that the attorney had remained silent.

* * * * *

The board then held a brief meeting. Taylor and Coleman joined Stackhouse in the hall and, after general comments about how things seemed to have gone,

Coleman left, saying he would be in touch with Taylor the next day. Ten minutes later members of the board left and St. Clair joined Taylor and Stackhouse. It now was near midnight and Taylor said he and St. Clair would return Stackhouse to his hotel.

When they arrived there, Taylor and St. Clair suggested that Stackhouse join them for a drink. The attorney was reluctant but the two were insistent, and they entered the cocktail lounge. A group of seven persons was sitting at two tables drawn together and when the three entered, several of the seven raised their hands and gestured. The three joined the party and Taylor and St. Clair introduced Stackhouse to seven members of the medical staff who had been waiting for their arrival.

In the conversation that followed for more than half an hour, the physicians told Stackhouse that Dr. Lee was a "menace" because he performed procedures that were unnecessary and that he had sexual problems that were manifested by his extraordinary interest in the clitoris. They made many other comments about Dr. Lee, none of which were favorable. The physicians also said that many more members of the medical staff shared their low opinion of the surgeon and hoped to see him gone from the hospital. They pressed St. Clair to tell them what he thought the board would do, based on the hearing.

St. Clair artfully dodged making a prediction. Taylor also declined to give one. The physicians turned to Stackhouse. He told them that if the board declined to take any major action against Dr. Lee, it would be their fault and that they, more than the board, would be responsible for his continuing presence at the hospital. He emphasized the impact on the board that the other physicians' testimony had provided for Dr. Lee. He then rose and made an abrupt exit. The physicians, and even St. Clair and Taylor, were disturbed by his comments.

The board members who participated in the hearing met five days later. There was considerable discussion, but no decision was forthcoming. The board met again a week later and, at that session, two positions were crystalized. The first was that although the charges against Dr. Lee had essentially been established, they were relatively minor and no more than an admonition or warning letter was appropriate. The second was that even if the failure to complete each record or to enter indications on each record was a minor matter in itself, the cumulative effect was serious enough for a more harsh disciplinary action. The Executive Committee members who were privy to information that had not been brought out at the hearing were a substantial part of the group taking this latter position. The board agreed to meet again in several days to take a final vote.

Meanwhile, at the hospital, each day that passed with no board action appeared to enhance Dr. Lee's stature considerably. He was abrasive with Taylor and other hospital employees and the list of his incomplete charts grew. Taylor told St. Clair what was happening and pressed him to get the board to make a decision that would restore some sense of discipline.

At the third board meeting after the hearing, a motion was made that Dr. Lee's appointment and all privileges at the hospital be suspended indefinitely. During the debate it was evident that some members of the board were in favor of the motion as introduced, others wanted a suspension for a definite time—the period most frequently mentioned was 15 to 30 days—and several urged merely admonishing the surgeon. Eventually, the question was called and the vote was 9 to 8 in favor of the motion to suspend Dr. Lee indefinitely. One of the board members then suggested that the vote on the motion be made unanimous. This was rejected by three members who said that under no circumstances could they go along with such severe disciplinary action.

The board, which had met without Taylor present, left the room and St. Clair informed the administrator of the decision. Taylor prepared a letter that he had delivered by hand to Dr. Lee announcing the board's action and informing the surgeon that he had until the following Monday to make arrangements for the continued care of his patients then in the hospital. No statement of facts found by the board supporting its decision to suspend Dr. Lee was considered, let alone prepared, and no transcript of the hearing was available to the board during any of its deliberations.

The next morning the hospital was served with a copy of an order to show cause why a preliminary injunction to prevent implementation of the suspension should not be issued, with a hearing set for the following Monday morning before Judge Jacob Roth of the local district court. Taylor immediately called Coleman and arranged for the legal papers to be hand-carried to the hospital's attorney. That night Coleman, Taylor, and St. Clair met to determine a course of action. The court reporter hired by the hospital by this time had completed the transcript of the hearing. Coleman prepared for the proceeding on Monday by gathering various hospital documents, the transcript of the hearing, and the documentary evidence that had been introduced. Taylor and St. Clair agreed to be in court.

* * * * *

At the appointed time Dr. Lee and Lewis, and Coleman, Taylor, and St. Clair appeared in Judge Roth's courtroom. The preliminary injunction, if issued, would restrain Taylor, the hospital board, and the hospital corporation from interfering with Dr. Lee's opportunity to care for his patients in the hospital or with his admission of new patients as their needs demanded.

Judge Roth asked Lewis to explain what had occurred at the hospital leading to the decision to discipline Dr. Lee. The attorney described the proceeding. The one-sided nature of his description left Coleman very upset. Judge Roth then asked Coleman to give his version and the hospital's counsel, referring to a number of passages in the transcript, sought to make clear the grounds that had led the board to make its decision and the evidence that had been put before it.

At this point Judge Roth asked counsel for both sides to join him in chambers. When they were together, the judge asked Coleman whether there was any way to resolve this controversy without the court's having to make a decision on granting a preliminary injunction against the hospital and, at the same time, accommodating the institution's interest.

Coleman replied that the board had labored long and hard through the hearing and three meetings to decide what, if any, sanction was to be imposed. It was his belief that the hospital's position was that it would not agree to any resolution or controversy without effective disciplinary action. Judge Roth then asked Lewis how much of a sanction Dr. Lee would be willing to accept as part of a settlement arrangement. The attorney said Dr. Lee felt that his failures, to the extent they might have been established by evidence at the hearing, were strictly matters of paper work and did not indicate any unsatisfactory professional performance.

Judge Roth asked Coleman for a copy of the hearing transcript made by the hospital's reporter. Lewis objected on the basis that he had not reviewed the transcript for accuracy, but the judge dismissed his objection, saying that he was looking for a way to resolve the matter quickly, if at all possible. While both attorneys sat in chambers, Judge Roth skimmed through the transcript.

After half an hour, during which Lewis and Coleman discussed between themselves the possibility of reaching an arrangement that would satisfy both the hospital and Dr. Lee, Judge Roth said he had a proposal to offer both sides:

Dr. Lee would continue to have his appointment and clinical privileges but he would not admit any additional patients to the hospital until he completed all incomplete records. Further, Judge Roth would lecture Dr. Lee in chambers about his failings as indicated by the transcript, and obtain his agreement to function within the state hospital licensing agency standards and the hospital's policies and procedures. On that basis, the court would refuse to grant the preliminary injunction because the relief was not necessary, the hospital having agreed to allow Dr. Lee's continued practice there. Lewis and Coleman were charged with discussing this proposal with their clients immediately.

Both Taylor and St. Clair were unhappy with the judicial intervention but Coleman urged them to accept the proposal. He said that, in his opinion, it was likely that Judge Roth would restrain the hospital from enforcing the suspension pending a full judicial hearing. While it was possible to appeal a preliminary injunction under some circumstances, the likelihood of success on appeal in advance of a full hearing, even if an appeal could be taken, was very slight.

Meanwhile, Lewis was attempting to win Dr. Lee's acceptance. The surgeon agreed to complete the records before admitting new patients but said he was very concerned about what Judge Roth might say to him. He did not want to accept an admonition from the judge because he believed he had done nothing improper of a professional nature.

Eventually, both attorneys were able to gain the agreement of their clients. With both attorneys, Taylor, St. Clair, and Dr. Lee present in chambers, Judge Roth stated his understanding that an agreement had been reached and asked the attorneys to prepare an order dismissing, with prejudice, the request for a preliminary injunction.

Judge Roth then began to lecture Dr. Lee. He told the surgeon he was very fortunate that the carelessness and arrogance he had displayed with regard to legitimate matters of hospital regulation had not brought him greater difficulty than already existed. The judge said he had some concern about Dr. Lee's professional reliability and mental balance because of the procedures around the clitoris, particularly since they apparently were taking place without the consent or prior knowledge of the patients. When Dr. Lee attempted to interrupt, Judge Roth silenced him with waves of the hand. He finished his lecture by saying:

"I am giving you a break, and it is the last one you will get from this court. If these good citizens from Community Hospital ever curb you again, and you come to this court for help, I want you to know that almost anything they want to do with you will be all right with me. You had better consider this as the last chance you will have in this county to straighten yourself out."

Turning to Taylor and St. Clair, Judge Roth said he was very pleased that the hospital had disciplined Dr. Lee. However, because he believed that it is possible for people to reform, and that a professional person such as a physician had the intelligence to understand what he was called upon to do by virtue of the standards of professional practice, he felt that more severe disciplinary action would serve no particular purpose. Having finished his admonitory remarks, Judge Roth said Dr. Lee might as well get back to taking care of his patients and Taylor to running the hospital, and that he would sign the necessary papers to complete the court's disposition of the matter.

* * * * *

Six months later Dr. Lee had achieved a much improved record at the hospital. He was performing far fewer sterilizations, there was no evidence that he was continuing to release adhesions around the clitoris, and he rarely had more than one or two tardy records when the lists of incomplete charts were posted. He avoided any contact with Taylor and Taylor had no particular reason to seek involvement with him.

During that six months, Dr. Lee and his wife were divorced. This appeared to improve his behavior and conduct toward hospital employees, particularly females, considerably. The director of nursing had not received any complaints about advances or physical touchings by Dr. Lee; whether they still took place was another matter, but there were no complaints.

St. Clair and other members of the board were quite pleased with the result. Dr. Lee had straightened out and there had not been exposure to the general public of the problems within the hospital to adversely affect the institution's reputation or its fund drive. Few persons in the community were even aware of the controversy.

Taylor believed he had been supported by the ultimate resolution of the dispute. The revising of the corporate bylaws and the medical bylaws still was dragging on and the administrator was concerned that at some time in the future another disciplinary problem would arise that would require taking prompt and effective action, but neither specific grounds for action nor a procedure to follow had yet been established by hospital documents.

Commentary

Three of the many matters in this case study are the subjects of this commentary: (1) the failure to have up-to-date hospital and medical staff documents; (2) the setting forth of grounds for disciplinary action and obtaining evidence to support charges; and (3) the response to judicial intervention.

1.

As the facts indicate clearly, after an initial determination that Dr. Lee was a problem physician, and after review of the hospital and medical staff documents then in effect, the board and administration both were well aware that there was a substantial need to revise the bylaws and regulations in the light of the then current needs, based on regulatory standards and the desire to reduce inhibitions to taking disciplinary action when it was appropriate.

Nevertheless, a year and a half elapsed during which bylaws revision was neglected for reasons not fully apparent from the case study but that can be assumed to include the absence of a specific charge to a committee or working group to proceed, with a stated time limit. The absence of a clearer statement of grounds for disciplinary action, other than "for cause," tended to inhibit decisiveness by the board. Community also was faced with the need to structure procedures to reduce the possibility of successful challenge by Dr. Lee on some sort of a due process issue in the event of a hospital decision adverse to him.

The absence of document provisions serves as a drag upon the taking of action when appropriate. Furthermore, the lack of suitable documents can create difficulty in meeting requirements of the Joint Commission on Accreditation of Hospitals and, in some states, it can lead to problems with the state hospital licensing agency. Findings of deficiencies in a review or survey process may lead the regulatory body to believe the hospital either is slovenly or is in the midst of some kind of internal crisis that prevents completion of the document revision process.

There are numerous sources of guidance for drafting modern hospital corporate bylaws, medical staff bylaws, and rules and regulations. These are readily available and can help reduce the burden on the committee or working group charged with the drafting task.

A realistic view must be taken of the time necessary to accomplish a revision of corporate and medical staff bylaws. The corporate bylaws revision, which is solely the responsibility of the board, assisted by staff, should be accomplished ordinarily within three or four months, once the decision has been made to undertake a comprehensive rewriting.

A list of basic changes that are believed advisable or necessary on subjects such as corporate membership, board composition, powers of the board in relation to the membership if the entity is a membership corporation, and other structural matters should be prepared. Several small working groups can be constituted to solicit opinions on various issues and to prepare recommendations based on the information gathered. There may be substantial areas of controversy that do not lend themselves to simple solutions. However, by clarifying the range of opinion on specific issues, the opportunity is created to crystalize the questions so that votes may be taken on the specific language of particular provisions.

The process for revision of medical staff bylaws tends to be longer and more complicated. The major drafting responsibility ordinarily is given to the medical staff. The extensive demands on physician time often prolong the process because of scheduling difficulties. In addition, the revision must take into consideration not only what the medical staff desires but also what the board will accept.

It often is useful to establish a small working group that leaves the legal details of drafting to the hospital attorney and focuses on substantive matters of bylaws content. For example, medical staff members should make the preliminary decisions concerning the categories of staff, whether and to what extent there should be specific language concerning provisional status for new members, voting privileges, committee responsibilities, election of staff officers (including officers of the entire staff and department chairmen), and the many other subjects that must be considered. The medical staff members should not burden themselves with drafting final language; their emphasis should be upon articulating what they believe to be desirable and communicating it to the person(s) actually doing the writing.

There must be some contact with representatives of the hospital board to ascertain the range of provisions it is likely to accept. Medical staff bylaws ordinarily cannot become effective until approved by both the medical staff and the board. It is helpful for the governing board, at the time this revision process begins, to prepare a list of the subjects it seeks to have covered. This would include topics not in the existing document as well as subjects for change. Board guidance to the drafting group usually is essential and can reduce unproductive efforts.

Even with an efficient drafting system, it is rare that the process is accomplished in less than a year, and a medical staff or board should not be particularly disheartened if it takes 18 months. While it always is possible to amend specific provisions of the medical staff bylaws relatively rapidly in response to a specific problem, a full-scale revision considers a great variety of subjects, many of which may require extensive changes in the current document. A major revision ordinarily should not be necessary more than every four or five years unless there has been an important, substantive revision of the Joint Commission standards or other pertinent regulatory material that imposes new requirements on the medical staff with respect to organization and procedures.

Returning to the case of Dr. Lee, the failure to have appropriate documents, while inhibiting prompt action to some extent, did not foreclose the eventual decisive action by the board. Based on the facts in this case, it is unlikely that at the time the situation existed a court would have found an absence of procedural due process in the handling of Dr. Lee, even in a state that had taken a liberal view on the rights of physicians in medical staff appointment and disciplinary controversies.

Today, the procedures established by Coleman and Stackhouse probably would not pass muster in states where the courts review procedures in more than a cursory manner. For example, the members of the Executive Committee of the board who became the body that decided to commence disciplinary action against Dr. Lee were privy to considerable evidence that was not introduced at the hearing. An argument might well be made successfully that they could not participate as objective members of the hearing and decision-making body because it would be difficult, if not impossible, for them to ignore the information they had received from Taylor, the administrator, and from items in the Lee file that were presented for their consideration.

Another due process consideration stemming from the ad hoc procedures related to the role of Coleman, the hospital attorney. In the preliminary stages he served as legal adviser to the board's Executive Committee. Then he took on the responsibility of drafting the charges and presenting the evidence to support them at the hearing. The argument could be made that the roles of board adviser and prosecutor, if that be the proper term, must be kept separate and filled by different attorneys.

Finally, as to due process in the conduct of the hearing itself, guidance was not provided to St. Clair, the board president, in his role as presiding officer. Because of the manner in which the litigation was concluded, and because of the failure to bring certain charges against Dr. Lee, close questions of admissibility of evidence truly did not arise. In more complicated proceedings it may be essential that a legally trained individual either preside or be available to counsel the presiding officer in order to avoid error that might be viewed by the court in subsequent litigation as substantial enough to require another hearing before disciplinary sanctions against the physician might be invoked.

2.

The hospital to some extent was fortunate that Dr. Lee had such a range of apparently unacceptable performances that the failure to present certain charges that might have been brought did not eliminate ample bases for taking disciplinary action. The decision to limit the charges was made because of the stated inability to obtain members of the medical staff to testify as to Dr. Lee's deviations from accepted medical practice, on the assumption that such charges therefore could not be substantiated. However, it always is possible to investigate the possibility, when members of the medical staff refuse to participate as expert witnesses, of obtaining evidence of the standard of appropriate medical practice from physicians at other hospitals in the area, or at a medical school, who would be willing to testify. Stackhouse, who supposedly was expert in medical staff matters, should have suggested specific ways to develop necessary expert testimony.

Furthermore, Coleman did not conduct an independent investigation of the possibility of obtaining evidence on Dr. Lee's behavior with members of the nursing service. While Taylor said the nurses were unwilling to participate in any proceeding against the surgeon, it is the attorney's function, once given the responsibility of preparing a case involving physician discipline, to personally evaluate the availability of evidence and, based on that determination, prepare the draft of charges for final decision within the hospital. Some hospital employees, speaking in confidence to an attorney, can be prevailed upon by that individual to come forward and provide testimony about such conduct, even though they express unwillingness to do so to a member of the hospital administration.

Concerning the failure to obtain consent for the clitoral area procedures performed on older women patients, and the question of fact relating to such procedures upon younger females, Coleman did not initiate any independent investigation of the possibility of supporting such charges. Rather, he sought to establish a minimum case, for which the evidence was relatively simple to obtain. Undoubtedly, questions of time, in view of the desire of Taylor, St. Clair, and the others to bring about prompt resolution of the problem, mitigated against taking a substantial period to conduct a painstaking investigation of all conduct to determine the full range of charges that might be brought.

Nevertheless, while Coleman's performance might be deemed satisfactory, given his inexperience in hospital medical staff matters and because the Lee case occurred before medical staff law blossomed as it has now, it might be questioned whether Judge Roth would have proposed the agreement he did if a transcript with evidence on the incidents with the nurses and other possible charges had been before him.

3.

There also is the question of how a hospital should respond to judicial intervention in a medical discipline case. Judge Roth, undoubtedly for the best of motives, sought to contain or settle the controversy rather than have it proceed further in litigation. There are many instances in which judges, when presented with petitions for equitable relief in strikes and other disputes, adopt a role of a mediator rather than solely a judicial officer. This is not necessarily inappropriate.

Nevertheless, the serious question exists as to how readily a hospital should bow to a settlement that results in a modest disciplinary action such as that in the case study. Evidently, the hospital was willing to take half or less of the loaf with the hope that the problem would be solved. Dr. Lee's attorney was able not only to save his client litigation expense but also to maintain his medical staff relationship as long as he refrained from further inappropriate conduct. Fortunately, Dr. Lee did reform, at least for the six months immediately following his day in court.

When the hospital has gone through the often arduous process of instituting a proceeding against a physician for serious reasons and, particularly, where the potential for success in litigation is great, judicial pressure to agree to a settlement should be resisted. Succumbing to it may be ill advised unless the hospital is confident that its purposes have been served. At the minimum, the hospital in the Lee matter should have required continuing judicial oversight over the surgeon's conduct.

Although Judge Roth took a strong position in his lecture to Dr. Lee, he again might have played the role of mediator or conciliator if the surgeon had appeared before him again. Coleman might have proposed that Judge Roth impose specific, objective standards for Dr. Lee's performance for some fixed period of time through an order that would have provided for immediate imposition of the suspension if the physician did not conform to them. For example, an order could include specification of the only acceptable grounds for sterilization, specific consent requirements, and details of medical record maintenance as standards to which Dr. Lee would have to conform. In essence, the judge could have granted the injunction to Dr. Lee, subject to its being lifted immediately on any evidence of departures from required performance. Judge Roth also had the power to require Dr. Lee to post bond that would subject him to potential financial loss.

Finally, it is possible that Dr. Lee's failures and misconduct before the litigation concluded in Judge Roth's court might be ignored as irrelevant or discounted by a judge in a later proceeding in which the surgeon challenged the disciplinary action against him in view of the settlement to which the hospital had agreed.

Case 6

Compassionate Death?

PERSONAE

Don Aarum, associate administrator of St. Luke's Hospital
Amy Austin, wife of the dying patient
Douglas Austin, the dying patient
Dr. Ahmad Bahari, neurologist on the Austin case
Jane Blanton, R.N., East Wing nursing supervisor
Dr. Andrew Boxer, director of medical education
Dr. Paul Browning, head of ICU
Dr. Joseph Cahn, director of anesthesia
Dr. Thomas Capwright, surgeon
Sister Danelle, legislative panelist
Don Doar, hospital house counsel
Bishop Wright Donaldson, chairman of hospital board
Margaret Doney, R.N., on Austin case
Peter Drury, district attorney
Dr. William Ensing, third-year resident, protagonist
J. Archer Hood, hospital's outside counsel
Jack Latole, hospital administrator
Colleen O'Meara, director of nursing
Ed Spolit, a hospital pharmacist
Dr. Edwin Williams, hospital chief of staff

What was to be a most eventful day began uneventfully for most of those involved. Dr. William Ensing characteristically forced himself out of bed at 5:45 A.M. after five hours of fitful sleep. Yesterday had been the sixth straight 12-hour day and today looked to be no different. Dr. Ensing was nearing completion of his third year of family practice residency at St. Luke's Hospital and for the last 10 days had been pulling service on the obstetrical unit. The hours were a marked change from the time demanded in the Department of Medicine, where he had spent the previous four months.

Jack Latole also was up early, as was his custom. He had mapped out his plans late in the afternoon of the previous day as he had finalized travel arrangements to the state capital for a legislative committee meeting of the state hospital association. Latole, in his seventh successful year as administrator of St. Luke's, had his usual reservations about leaving the hospital "unattended," for Don Aarum, his associate administrator, was attending one of his many seminars. The director of nursing, Colleen O'Meara, had spent the better part of the previous morning with Latole and he was fairly confident that she could manage in his two-day absence.

Amy Austin did not really wake up this Tuesday morning for she had not really slept. She had spent all Monday night, as well as all day Sunday, at St. Luke's, tending to her painful vigil. Sleep, if it came at all, was in 20-minute spurts, ending in worry about Doug and the children, and fear for herself.

Douglas Austin did not notice the dawning of Tuesday any more than he had Monday or Sunday. Saturday morning was the last sunrise he had appreciated as he opened his Texaco station at 6 A.M. On Saturday he worked only until 10 in the morning because he was due at St. Luke's at 11 for his every-third-week progress analysis. Doug had known for four months that he had a brain tumor, for three months that it was malignant, and for the last five weeks that there was a slow pattern of growth. Because of its location, surgery was not possible, and the best hope for a course of chemotherapy was to retard its development and extend his already shortened life. His sudden lapse into unconsciousness in midmorning Saturday, shortly before his appointment, ended even that hope.

Bishop Wright Donaldson, not unlike Amy Austin, had slept fitfully Monday night, as his wife pointedly noted. All day Monday he had presided and politicked at the chaotic quarterly meeting of the synod. Abortion was the topic of both floor and anteroom discussion, and only with the bishop's persuasive forcefulness did the synod take a dramatic change of direction and proclaim a strong position in opposition to abortion. The cost in personal friendship, the quiet anger of his wife, and perhaps parishoners' defections to other synods lay heavily on his mind as he tried to think positively of the two days of unscheduled activities ahead of him.

* * * * *

Following the Tuesday morning conference in the Intensive Care Unit, Dr. Ahmad Bahari put out a page for Dr. Ensing, then on his third cup of coffee in the employees' lounge. Dr. Bahari was a most conservative neurologist by Dr. Ensing's appraisal. He surprised Dr. Ensing with the report that the senior staff had recommended transferring Austin out of ICU and that Dr. Bahari concurred. Dr. Ensing knew well of Austin's status and prognosis because he was the first doctor Amy Austin called on Saturday. ICU had but two empty beds, Austin was stable and slowly deteriorating, and thus the conclusion was reached that transfer to a private room was in order. Dr. Bahari, who knew Austin only slightly after just four visits, and Amy not at all, was relieved that Dr. Ensing had developed good rapport with the family during his tour on the medical and neurology service. Passing news of the imminence of death was not a task that Dr. Bahari performed well, and he knew it.

Amy Austin had the mixed feelings of despair and relief as Dr. Ensing gently but clumsily explained her husband's status and the details of the transfer. A private room would almost be a blessing following the bright lights and technical coldness of the ICU. A sense of the rapid approach of Doug's death was present but almost muffled by the bustle of the patient cart and transport process to the fourth floor. Amy never was more than five feet from Doug as the nurse and aides moved the passive man from the unit, to the cart, to the elevator, and finally to the quiet of Room 403.

Dr. Ensing, who at the call of the director of OB, rushed back to the labor room where two mothers-to-be were in need of his attention, quickly absorbed himself in the immediate tasks at hand. In his years of residency at St. Luke's, fate, luck, or coincidence had limited his exposure to the dying process and the three patients he had watched die his first year also were the last three. Dealing directly with family at such times was something he felt able to do but the experience had eluded him. He wondered how his inexperience must have looked to Amy Austin, a quiet but strong woman whom he had come to know fairly well during her husband's many visits to the outpatient department in the last several months.

It was noon before Dr. Ensing was able to complete his OB duties and visit the Austins in 403. Lunch was forgotten as he saw the family crowded into the corner of the room. All eyes were averted from the bed where Doug lay fitful and restless. His parents and sister, as well as the two near-adolescent Austin boys, had arrived together shortly before Dr. Ensing, and the mutual discomfort of all was apparent as small talk was exchanged. Doug's increasingly labored breathing added to the strain of the setting.

Amy, with subdued control, quickly turned to Dr. Ensing, "Can anything be done to ease his breathing and make him more comfortable?" she asked.

Searching his memory of senior year, Dr. Ensing answered with deliberation that repositioning Austin might help. Out of earshot of the children, he explained, "We could position a support below his neck and shoulders to ease the breathing. However, if we do, it will most likely extend the process somewhat."

"How much longer will it be?" Austin's sister asked quickly.

"Dr. Bahari wasn't sure, but it should be early afternoon at most," he replied.

"Do what you can, but please make him as comfortable as possible," Amy quickly added, followed by a concurring nod from Doug's mother.

Dr. Ensing encouraged the family to move to the solarium, and all but Amy quickly agreed. After everyone else had left, she quietly asked to stay with Doug for the duration. Dr. Ensing acceded to the request and paused to hear her further feelings before he left to look for a nurse and more pillows. Both were found together, as he met Margaret Doney, R.N., around the corner. A quick explanation brought two firm pillows and the aid of Nurse Doney at once.

Margaret Doney, although only two years out of school, obviously attended the process of dying more often than Dr. Ensing. Still, experience in this area is not a teacher to everyone, and she shared his discomfort as they approached the straining Douglas Austin. The young doctor now was much more comfortable in talking with Amy about the options.

"If we do nothing, the breathing will become more and more of a strain on Doug," he said, as they talked at the head of the bed. "Dr. Bahari said, and I think he's right, that the natural process, if he remains as he is, will soon put substantial pressure on his chest and lungs. I know it is hard to accept and watch, but it would bring on death fairly quickly."

"How?" Amy asked.

"By a process of suffocation."

Amy's composure almost left her as they discussed the process of raising Doug's shoulders and neck to allow his head to lie off the back of the pillow, easing the strain.

"I've been with several families in cases like these," Nurse Doney added, "and it can be hard on the family. Mr. Austin appears to be strong, so his death could be long and difficult."

The choice was left to Amy and she quickly avoided a long-drawn-out decision by urging Dr. Ensing and Nurse Doney to ease the breathing with pillows.

* * * * *

That afternoon, 5:30 came soon for Dr. Ensing as his assigned tour for the day ended. Two women were in labor, but another third-year resident volunteered to cover, knowing well that Dr. Ensing had Room 403 and the Austins on his mind. Dr. Ensing was surprised to find Nurse Doney in the room when he arrived, since she already had worked the day shift. A shortage of staff and her interest in helping ease the process to an end provided a ready answer to his query.

She told Dr. Ensing that Doug had continued in a strained manner, and the heavy sound of breathing filled the room. All of the family but Amy had left the hospital, ready to return upon her call.

I've tried to reach Dr. Bahari three times but he hasn't called in,'' Nurse Doney said. ''It seems that a muscle relaxant might ease his breathing somewhat.''

Dr. Ensing tried to reach Dr. Bahari himself and, finding no answer at home, called Dr. Paul Browning, the head of ICU, at his house and explained the status of the case. Dr. Browning, knowing Austin's case only slightly because of his late arrival at the ICU conference, could offer little direction. Dr. Browning was not directly in charge of the care of this individual and was very reluctant to order any care for Dr. Bahari's patient. He and Dr. Bahari had had several sharp differences in recent months over resuscitator patients and Dr. Browning was not about to assume direction of this, one of the few cases where he thought Dr. Bahari had reached a decisive and correct decision.

''The process should take care of itself soon,'' he said. ''I would do nothing but keep the family comfortable and be as supportive as you can.''

''Should I give him any relaxants?'' Dr. Ensing asked.

''I wouldn't, but use your own judgment,'' Dr. Browning said. He knew Dr. Ensing slightly as a bright, if somewhat too conscientious, resident, and he liked him.

''Thanks,'' thought Dr. Ensing as he hung up and gazed down the hall. The sound of Austin's strained breathing could be heard through the nearly closed door fours room away. Nurse Doney came out of the door, closed it gently behind her, and, lost in thought and drained, walked past him without apparently seeing him. She did not cry often or easily but she brushed several tears aside as she entered Nursing Conference Room B. Dr. Ensing picked up the phone and called Pharmacy.

''One hundred cc anectine IV for Mr. Austin in 403.''

''Anectine?'' Ed Spolit asked in genuine surprise. In his years as a pharmacist at St. Luke's, he couldn't recall anectine's being ordered to a floor because it was used almost exclusively in the OR and ER as an anesthetic.

''Yes, we have a patient who was transferred from ICU and I need a muscle relaxant,'' Dr. Ensing replied. He was mildly irritated at the inquiry, as again he felt that Pharmacy questioned too many orders.

Twenty minutes later both the anectine and East Wing Nursing Supervisor Jane Blanton arrived at Four East at the same time. Nurse Doney logged in the pharmacy report as Ms. Blanton tried to think of a reason why anectine would be on the floor.

"Who's that for?" she asked Nurse Doney.

"Dr. Ensing is caring for a terminal patient of Dr. Bahari's and he needs a muscle relaxant to ease his breathing. I couldn't reach Dr. Bahari, but Dr. Ensing said he talked to Dr. Browning," the nurse answered.

"One cc too many of anectine and he'll be more than relaxed, he'll be dead," Ms. Blanton stated matter-of-factly. "Does Dr. Ensing know how to use that?"

"He told me he worked with Dr. Capwright in surgery for two weeks and was amazed at the effects of it in anesthesia," the nurse replied.

"I don't know. Keep me informed," Ms. Blanton said as she headed up to Five.

* * * * *

The arrival of 9:45 P.M. in Room 403 made Nurse Doney most uneasy. For the past hour, the vigil continued to be painful as Austin subconsciously called upon his tremendous strength to continue his tortured breathing. Three times Dr. Ensing had directed her to administer anectine IV, the first two times 5 cc each and the last, at 9:30, 10 cc. Each was followed shortly by a sudden easing in Austin's trial, only to have him soon revert to his loud struggle.

The death rattle had been present for the past half hour. Amy Austin's tears were gone, her eyes drawn from the strain and lack of sleep.

"Can't you help him again?" she asked Dr. Ensing. "He seems to be hurting so."

"We can, but each time we do, we shorten the process," he answered thoughtfully."

"Please! Please do something, do anything!" she urged.

"Margaret, 20 cc," he directed the nurse.

"I can't," she said. "I just can't." Dr. Ensing took the anesthetic and through the IV in Austin's ankle, added 20 cc at 9:52 P.M. Douglas Austin died at 9:53 P.M.

* * * * *

The note passed to Jack Latole the next morning caught him off guard, for though he was presiding at the committee meeting in the state capital, his mind was on his daughter and her choice of Idaho State as a college next year. He couldn't even estimate the number of miles or how to get there.

"Call your attorney at his office. It's urgent." All of his calls were "urgent," the St. Luke's administrator thought. The last urgent one had involved a pheasant hunting trip to Nebraska.

"Take over, I'll be right back," he told Sister Danelle, who was sitting on his right.

"We may have a mercy killing on our hands," J. Archer Hood, the attorney for St. Luke's, said in his third sentence on the phone. "It seems that a resident may have deliberately overdosed a dying patient last night on Four East. The bishop is in town for the Executive Committee meeting tonight and he fell right into it while talking with Colleen this morning. Called me right away!"

"Who's the resident?" Latole asked.

"A fellow named Bill Ensing. In family practice, second or third year," the attorney replied.

The name was only vaguely familiar to Latole, for with 950 beds and three residency programs, he never met all the residents. After obtaining more particulars from the thorough Hood, Latole hung up and began planning an immediate return home. Two phone calls followed: one to Colleen O'Meara, the director of nursing, to verify and complete the details, and the other to chairman of the board, Bishop Donaldson, at his motel. After talking with his chairman, Latole knew that the legislative committee meeting would have to be closed by Sister Danelle, not him.

* * * * *

Colleen O'Meara was in conference with the chief of staff, Dr. Edwin Williams, when Latole called. Jane Blanton also was present and the details not furnished by Hood were provided by the three conferees. The day already had been long, for this Wednesday morning had been filled with meetings involving the death of Douglas Austin and the procedures in Room 403 the night before. Dr. Williams spent half an hour on the phone with Dr. Browning, the head of the ICU, and finally tracked down Dr. Bahari, the ICU neurologist, in Kansas City for another hour-long phone conference. Hood had been at the hospital at 9 A.M. following Ms. O'Meara's call at 7. Don Doar, newly hired house counsel for St. Luke's, was greeted with the facts on his arrival at 8:45. Thus, by the time Latole called at 11, Ms. O'Meara was "conferenced out."

"I'm still trying to decide if we have a residency problem, a medical staff problem, a criminal problem, or no problem at all," Dr. Williams mused. "Whatever we call it, should the press pick it up, we've got one helluva P.R. problem," he added to no one in particular.

Dr. Williams, a general surgeon in his second year of a two-year term as chief of staff, had his own strong views on the passive/active euthanasia question. Even feeling strongly that more should be done for the definitely dying patient to terminate pain and perhaps shorten the dying process, Dr. Ensing's treatment had him upset.

Dr. Williams knew that the nature of Austin's condition was such that no pain was involved; rather, the "pain" was for those who waited and watched. Although not agreeing fully, he also knew of Bishop Donaldson's strong views against euthanasia and his consistently "pro-life" views on abortion. What he did not know was the attitude of the local district attorney and the possible publicity or political overtones of the situation. Although stories of "mercy killings" had been reported in other states, he could not recall any arising locally.

Dr. Williams was angry at Dr. Bahari, an anger he kept to himself; he also was slightly perturbed with Dr. Browning. Dr. Browning's lack of involvement and absence of direction to Dr. Ensing was somewhat understandable, given his previous run-ins with Dr. Bahari. But Dr. Bahari's failure to assume full charge of Austin's case, much less his allowing a resident from another service to fend for himself, was inexcusable. All of this had then been compounded by his unavailability for more than 24 hours. Then Pharmacy had sent anectine to the floor on the order of a resident! And right past an experienced nursing supervisor!

"All of the checks in the system shorted out," he thought.

* * * * *

Latole's full conference began at 3 P.M. and wound down at about 5:30. All the authorities were there: Bishop Donaldson, Dr. Williams, Hood, Doar, Ms. O'Meara, and Dr. Browning. They were visited briefly by Dr. Joseph Cahn, director of anesthesia, who provided clinical information regarding anectine, its uses, and its effects. Dr. Cahn firmly believed that the drug, while fast acting, could not possibly have moved through the system and paralyzed the respiratory muscles in the time recounted by Nurse Doney. Three to five minutes maybe, but not one. He did acknowledge that, given Austin's constitution and the dosage involved, it would have brought on paralysis and death.

Halfway through the meeting, Dr. Andrew Boxer, director of medical education, joined the group. He was able to fill in background details on Dr. Ensing. His analysis supported Dr. Browning's feelings that Dr. Ensing was a hard-working, intelligent, if somewhat overly conscientious, young physician. Dr. Boxer had counseled Dr. Ensing only last month about his tendency to get too close to his patients, becoming a bit too involved with them and their feelings. He had urged Dr. Ensing to work harder at walking the line between aloofness and overinvolvement in order to retain both the objectivity and compassion needed in the practice of medicine, particularly if he was to be in family practice.

"You mean you urged him to be more distant, more technical, with his patients?" Bishop Donaldson asked with some incredulity. "It seems to me that we should be doing just the opposite!"

"It's a matter of balance," Dr. Williams interjected. "Neither melodramatic compassion nor a sterile technical approach is healthy as a manner of practice, but rather a blending of both. Some people are born with the ability to do it well, some learn through experience, and, unfortunately, some never master the ability to walk the line, to achieve that blending."

The meeting was broken by short spells of silence as the attendees struggled with the issues. As time wore on, these spells came more often and became more uncomfortable. Each individual began to inquire of Hood and Doar, the hospital attorneys, as to their legal choices and concerns. Doar, nine months out of law school, was inclined to believe that the matter was best left to the educational process of the residency program, and stated his views to that effect. Hood, having exposure to a criminal practice and from a consultation with an associate in his firm with prior experience in the district attorney's office, was not convinced that the case was free of criminal law implications.

Hood summarized the options, ranging from a heart-to-heart talk with Dr. Ensing and Nurse Doney to a full report to the district attorney. The options between the spectrum's ends included the possibility of transfer or termination of Dr. Ensing's residency or employment and the same for Nurse Doney; various reprimands for the other physicians and employees; discussions with the various state licensing boards; and notice to the hospital's malpractice insurance carrier to cover the remote possibility of a complete change of attitude by Amy Austin or someone acting on behalf of her now fatherless children.

More thought and discussion resulted in a decision to meet with Dr. Ensing. No one at this point had seen him except Doar. It was not only Dr. Ensing's day off but he had been up until 2:30 A.M. with the Austin family and, reportedly, was both exhausted and drained by the ordeal. Doar had spoken with him in person in the early afternoon—he had come to know Dr. Ensing from occasional racquetball matches. The fact that Doar was aware of Austin's death compounded Dr. Ensing's anxiety when he was requested to join the meeting.

* * * * *

The meeting with Dr. Ensing did not go as anticipated. Hood and Dr. Williams had concurred beforehand and brought about a consensus that a conference with the district attorney was a must. Arrangements had been made to meet with him at 10 o'clock that night. The chief of staff also had concluded personally that Dr. Ensing had to go, the only questions being where, and whether the Board of Medical Examiners should be involved. He would deal with Drs. Bahari and Browning later.

Dr. Ensing's worries were apparent as he sat down with the group of two attorneys, the administrator, chief of staff, director of nursing, director of medical education, and chairman of the board who, to his further dismay, turned out to be a bishop. Dr. Boxer, who knew Dr. Ensing best of those present, said they wanted to hear from him the details of Austin's death so that hospital representatives who would be meeting later with the district attorney could be as informed as possible.

With no further urging than his own worries and concerns, Dr. Ensing began a recital of the details of his care for and relationship with Doug Austin and his family:

How he came to know them on outpatient clinic duty and had shared their initial moments of terror on the discovery of Doug's tumor and its eventual diagnosis; how he ended up as "their" doctor when the assigned physician failed to relate to their need for support and encouragement; how this resulted in his spending the last two days as, for all intents and purposes, the attending physician when none other was available or interested; how he extended Austin's life by repositioning him to aid his breathing (which also added a touch of macabre to the room); how Austin's physical strength prolonged his death by hours and added to the sounds and sensations of the dying process; how the ties between him and Nurse Doney and Amy Austin tightened in the late hours of the day, and were compounded by the physical exhaustion they all shared; how he had thought of anectine and how its use and effectiveness had been explained carefully to him by the anesthesiologist; how it was used for Austin; why and how Austin died as and when he did; and finally, how he believed that he intended not to kill him but that he did know that while anectine would ease the breathing somewhat, it clearly would shorten the dying process.

Dr. Ensing spoke uninterruptedly and undistracted by the tears that passed down his cheeks as he recreated the scenes of the last two days. As his chronology came to the point where he received the request to come to the meeting, his voice trailed off and stopped. Another of those uncomfortable silent spells fell over the group and ended with a gentle question or two from Dr. Williams and Bishop Donaldson. After Dr. Ensing was excused with words of encouragement, silence again filled the room.

* * * * *

The meeting with the district attorney, Peter Drury, beginning at 10:15 P.M. rather than at 10, was subdued and somewhat different from what had been intended when it was scheduled. Dr. Williams presented the facts to the attentive district attorney, speaking in a mixture of clinical and nonclinical terms, while leaving the impression that this mistake of judgment probably was not causal from a medical-legal standpoint.

"Do you plan on keeping him as a resident?" Drury asked when Dr. Williams concluded.

"Definitely, although we may allow him some time away and provide some counseling," Dr. Williams replied. "He is a good doctor and I think should overcome this and be the better for it."

Hood spoke guardedly in terms of causation, criminal intent and lack therof, and the medical expectations that Austin should have died Tuesday afternoon; how after 9 P.M. on Tuesday, the doctors present fully believed that death was always minutes away; how only Austin's unexpected strength upset their beliefs; why the pillow was positioned in the first place and why it was not removed until after he died.

* * * * *

Three days later, Hood received a two-page letter from Drury, summarizing the district attorney's analysis and setting forth his rationale that there was not sufficient evidence indicating that criminal activity had occurred. The letter was marked personal and confidential. The bottom indicated no carbon copies were distributed.

After returning from a two-day visit home, Dr. Ensing resumed coverage in maternity. Nurse Doney still was on leave of absence from Four East. That day Dr. Williams had spent a long and unpleasant half hour together with Drs. Bahari and Browning, going over the need both for professional relationships with attending staff members and controlled supervision of new additions and residents. Both were told that their professional relationship must improve between now and reappointment review.

Latole spent half of that Saturday reviewing architectural drawings with Aarum, his "visiting" associate administrator. Hood called and informed him of the letter from the district attorney, and Dr. Williams dropped in after his session with Drs. Bahari and Browning. Latole put in a call to Bishop Donaldson at noon to report on the architectural plans as well as to give him an update on the day's mail and meetings. The bishop was relieved to hear of the district attorney's letter but was still bothered with lingering feelings of uncertainty about the chain of events. He also was extremely irritated with the architect and his projections.

Commentary

The dying person, once the typical patient in American hospitals, engenders a variety of problems, as indicated in this case study. Modern medicine's role is to heal and cure, and the frustration in instances when a death is inevitable can be consuming.

For those involved in this actual incident, the return to their duties was not "business as usual" as the closing might indicate. The experience was emotionally traumatic for all involved for it brought into conscious consideration life-and-death choices, moral and legal concerns, and in-depth professional evaluations.

Could this "crisis" have been prevented or avoided? Perhaps, but maybe not. The demands on the health care system today make it almost a certainty that these types of situations will arise. Some lessons can be drawn from the case, however.

1.

The medical education process envisions supervised and directed clinical experience in the residency programs. On occasion, the degree of supervision designed into the programs is not achieved, as was the case in this situation. The unavailability of the attending physician without providing back-up, with the result that full responsibility for the patient fell upon a resident outside of his service, is a rarity and obviously not desirable.

2.

Entwined in this report is the clash of professional personalities that heightens the already existing reluctance of one physician, even if in a supervisory position such as a department chairman, to intervene in the case of another doctor's patient. Here it is even further aggravated by the lack of onsite consultation available to the resident.

3.

The requirement in the immediate review of the actions of the resident and nursing personnel, to attempt to enter their minds to determine Dr. Ensing's intent, was the most difficult aspect of the analysis of the incident. The district attorney's conclusion was, perhaps at that point in the process, the easiest to achieve. He had to determine both whether there were facts available to support a finding of criminal activity and whether the facts could be presented in a manner that could bring a conviction.

4.

The professional evaluation as to whether the course of treatment was appropriate from a medical standpoint was more difficult for it entered into the delicate area of medical-moral conduct. The concept of palliative care is in a state of evolution, and what is palliative to one may be euthanasia to another. Religious sponsorship of a hospital may further accentuate these concerns and intensify the decision-making and evaluation process.

5.

The observation by the chief of staff that the check system failed is worthy of note. Pharmacy and nursing today should not stand idly by in situations involving an apparently erroneous order or the inappropriate use of certain drugs or procedures. In situations where responsible medical intervention may be needed, it most likely will be precipitated by nursing service, or perhaps pharmacy, and personnel in those departments should know their responsibilities in this respect and should be supported when they initiate action, even if it may be incorrect on occasion.

6.

Most established medical care audit and review systems are not designed for analysis of this type of case. Had the facts been different and involved an attending staff member, it can only be conjectured whether the issue would have surfaced publicly and what course of action the review might have taken.

It is probable that these types of cases are rare but it is doubtful that they are unique to this institution. Accordingly, it would be beneficial to both medical and nursing personnel that educational and counseling conferences and, perhaps, on-call staff assistance be available to aid in the treatment of the dying patient as well as to help and support the immediate family.

Case 7

Telling It Like It Is

PERSONAE

Liz Carey, hospital patients' rights coordinator

Dr. Lyle English, chairman of the Departments of Psychiatry at both the hospital and the university

Dr. Arnold Fineman, hospital medical director

Franklin Hummer, hospital administrator

Dr. Alan Rosen, director of outpatient clinic in hospital's Department of Psychiatry and assistant professor of psychiatry at the university, protagonist

James Stoner, hospital house counsel

Dr. Alan Rosen, if asked, would openly attribute his successful career to his brilliant mind, his self-confidence, his quick wit, and his hard work. Indeed, his record throughout medical school and his residency in psychiatry supported his assessment of his qualities. Further, his rather bombastic and colorful personality made him attractive to the news media, to lawyers looking for an expert witness, to various research interests, and to patients. Yes, Dr. Rosen always prided himself in never avoiding controversy and in "telling it like it is!"

Upon completion of his residency, Dr. Rosen decided to begin his career in academic medicine. This choice would afford him the opportunity to conduct research, to publish, and to make a name for himself. He also knew that physicians in academia could nicely supplement their incomes through private patient care and consulting activities. He fully expected to be a professor and have a Cadillac before he reached the age of 40.

Dr. Rosen had been an assistant professor in psychiatry at a major university on the East Coast when he met and worked with Dr. Arnold Fineman. Dr. Fineman had won international acclaim through his books and teachings on innovative concepts in the assessment and delivery of specialized medical services. In 1974, he accepted a university professorship and the position as medical director of the University Hospital in a metropolitan area in the West. Dr. Fineman invited Dr. Rosen to join him as director of an outpatient clinic within the Department of Psychiatry, promising him first-class treatment and a bright future. Dr. Rosen gladly accepted because of the promise and because he had high regard and respect for Dr. Fineman's intelligence and shrewdness.

University Hospital is a free-standing nonprofit corporation with 647 inpatient beds and more than 300,000 outpatient visits per year. Eighty of the inpatient beds are assigned to the Department of Psychiatry, which also accounts for more than 50,000 of the outpatient visits annually. In terms of patient visits, the outpatient clinic directed by Dr. Rosen is the largest in the department.

As the name implies, University Hospital is affiliated, by agreement, with the local university. Therefore, with few exceptions, all members of the hospital medical staff also must hold faculty appointments in the university's School of Medicine. The recruitment and retention of medical staff members is a joint function of the hospital and the university. The affiliation agreement provides a rather elaborate procedure for accomplishing this process:

> Except as hereinafter provided, the Hospital agrees that it shall not appoint or reappoint a physician to its medical staff unless and until such individual has received an academic appointment in the School of Medicine of the University.
>
> Nominations for appointment to the Active Medical Staff shall originate in the Hospital in accordance with its bylaws. Notification of each nomination shall be submitted by the Hospital to the University. In each instance the Hospital shall submit information to the University sufficient for the University to evaluate the nominee for academic appointment. The President or his designee on behalf of the University shall then approve or disapprove the nominee's academic appointment. Action taken by the University on each suggested nomination shall be reported in writing within 45 days (after the date the information was submitted to the University) to the Governing Board of the Hospital with a copy to the Hospital's Chief Executive Officer.
>
> In the event of disapproval, the basis shall be submitted in writing to the Governing Board of the Hospital. If in the opinion of the Govern-

ing Board of the Hospital the requested appointment continues to be in the best interest of the Hospital and its patients, the Governing Board of the Hospital may request that the dispute be arbitrated by the Chairman of the Governing Board of the Hospital and the President of the University. It is understood and agreed that one possible result of the arbitration of a disputed appointment would be the election by the Governing Board of the Hospital to appoint the nominee to the Courtesy Staff without academic appointment. In no event will academic appointments be granted without recommendation by the Faculty and approval by the President in the case of tenured, and by the Provost, in the case of untenured appointments.

Termination by the University of the academic appointment of any member of the Hospital Active Staff will not take place without prior discussion with the Hospital Governing Board, since as stated above, with certain exceptions, all members of the Active Staff of the Hospital must have an academic appointment. Termination of tenured Faculty appointments are subject to tenure rules. Those of untenured Faculty are subject to University due process procedures.

If, in the opinion of the Governing Board, the retention of a physician on the Active Staff whose faculty appointment is to be terminated, is in the best interest of the Hospital and its patients, the Governing Board of the Hospital may request that the dispute be arbitrated by the Chairman of the Governing Board of the Hospital and the President of the University. It is understood and agreed that one possible result of the arbitration of a disputed termination would be the election by the Governing Board of the Hospital to retain the physician on the Medical Staff without academic appointment.

Due process procedures in the Hospital Medical Staff bylaws shall be used for Medical Staff appointments, reappointments, and terminations. Due process procedures in the University shall be used for granting of and changes in faculty appointments, reappointments, and terminations.

* * * * *

Dr. Rosen was appointed initially as an assistant professor and currently was under consideration for promotion to a tenured associate professorship. Members of the hospital medical staff who are full-time faculty members were responsible for direct patient care, teaching, and research. Clinical directors, such as Dr. Rosen, also had additional administrative and supervisory responsibilities for which they received special compensation. Although hospital medical staff members who were full-time faculty were considered employees of the university, they were subject to both hospital and university policies and procedures, including the hospital staff handbook, the medical staff bylaws, and the university handbook for faculty.

The key to Dr. Rosen's promotion would be the recommendation of his superior, Dr. Lyle English, chairman of both the hospital and university Departments of Psychiatry. Dr. English had worked at University Hospital and had been a faculty member at the university for 25 years. He was a native of the locality, where he had taken great pride in the community relationships he had established with patients, other physicians, and service agencies. Unlike many of his colleagues, he did not travel much and ensured that his nights and weekends were spent at home. He perceived himself as a senior clinical administrator with the patients' interests at heart. He had been a little suspicious about an increased emphasis on research since the arrival of Dr. Fineman.

For a number of reasons, Dr. Rosen and Dr. English had not been on the best of terms with each other almost since they first met. The newcomer openly criticized the department chairman for being indecisive and without significant academic credentials. On the other hand, Dr. English on several occasions expressed concern to Dr. Fineman about Dr. Rosen's unwillingness to follow directions and his perceived placement of self before patient care.

Several factors appeared to have brought their relationship to the boiling point. A few of Dr. English's associates had discussed with him the fact that Dr. Fineman considered Dr. Rosen to be his "fair-haired boy." Dr. English also felt that Dr. Fineman as medical director was too sympathetic to Dr. Rosen because he had recruited Dr. Rosen, and because Dr. Fineman seemed to like the favorable media attention his "protege" had brought to the hospital and to the university. A science writer from a local newspaper recently had run a series on Dr. Rosen's experience with the relationship between affective and cognitive disorders in women. Dr. Rosen also was pushing himself to complete his research and publications before the meeting of his academic promotion committee.

Although not so much of a concern to Dr. English, hospital administrations nationwide were putting constant pressure on their outpatient clinics to operate more efficiently since Blue Cross, Blue Shield, and Medicaid payments were not sufficient to meet the costs of providing the services. Partly as a response to this pressure, and partly to free more of his own time, Dr. Rosen structured his clinic in such a way that the patient primary care role now rested more with his nurse clinicians than when he arrived. Initial evaluations to determine whether patients would be accepted by the clinic, and analyses of continuing treatment, were provided by nurses or, to a more limited extent, by psychiatric residents.

Dr. Rosen authorized nurses to use his signature stamp on noncontrolled drug prescriptions and encouraged them to make routine and minor treatment follow-up changes on their own. They were permitted to propose diagnostic formulations and treatment plans to Dr. Rosen or other physician supervisors, including residents. Dr. Rosen had attempted to minimize the amount of his constant "hovering over the shoulder" supervision.

Although Dr. Rosen recognized his ultimate clinic supervisory responsibilities for evaluations, treatment plans, and continuing patient care, he admitted that the structure of his clinic deviated from physician-centered health care delivery, which was particularly prevalent in university teaching hospitals. His clinic did not accept patients who expressed a preference to see a psychiatrist exclusively and, when possible, referred them to private practitioners. Dr. Rosen believed that following the more traditional medical model approach would prevent the clinic from providing services to more than 400 patients at any time. Nor was he particularly concerned about the training of psychiatric residents assigned to his clinic who were openly critical of his heavy reliance on nurses.

* * * * *

Dr. English was aware of the structure of Dr. Rosen's clinic and of his supervisory style. Since he was concerned about the legal status of this approach, Dr. English asked the hospital's in-house legal counsel, James Stoner, for an opinion. After personally reviewing the situation with Dr. English and Dr. Rosen, Stoner advised both physicians in a memo stating, in essence, that:

1. The refusal to accept into the clinic a patient who desired a greater amount of direct physician care than Dr. Rosen was willing to provide, or who did not meet certain research design parameters, could be construed as a breach of the hospital's representations to the community and of the hospital's contractual agreements with Blue Cross, Blue Shield, Medicare, Medicaid, and federal/state governments in accepting Hill-Burton funds. Over the years, the hospital, as a nonprofit corporation, had been represented to the community as being responsive to the health care needs of the area's populace, regardless of patient race, creed, or religion. Thus, there was the potential for complaints from patients' rights groups. Stoner particularly emphasized the dangers of not providing care to a patient who was seriously ill. Further, hospital reimbursement agreements with private and public third party payers stressed broad patient service coverage with significant physician direction and supervision. He also mentioned the fraud and abuse aspects of billing third party payers for patient services that were not directed and supervised by physicians.
2. State law clearly mandated that only physicians could prescribe drugs and it did not matter whether or not they were controlled substances. State

law also prohibited the use of a stamp for the physician's signature on the prescription form. State law allowed licensed nurses only to administer, not prescribe, drugs.

3. There was significant movement in the state legislature to enact laws that would recognize expanded roles for licensed nurse practitioners and physician assistants, if qualified. However, Stoner noted that such legislation had yet to be passed.

4. State law permitted only physicians to be licensed to practice medicine. While the statutory definition of the practice of medicine was not very specific, the courts interpreted it fairly broadly in a manner to prevent other than licensed physicians from practicing. Stoner said the pending state legislation concerning licensed nurse practitioners and physician assistants would allow such persons to perform a limited number of medical practice acts but only under the supervision of a physician.

With all of these factors in mind, Stoner suggested that the hospital be cautious about the number of acts nonphysicians could perform without actual physician direction and involvement. Based on this advice, Dr. English met with Dr. Rosen and directed him to ensure that physicians evaluated patients and prescribed all medications for those receiving care in his clinic. He also asked Dr. Rosen to arrange for greater physician participation in the assessment, treatment plan development, delivery of care, and follow-up of patients. Dr. English confirmed these directions by sending Dr. Rosen a registered letter. He never before had communicated this way with one of his physicians but he hoped that this method would stress the importance of the message.

The meetings with Stoner and Dr. English had made Dr. Rosen angry, and upon receipt of the registered letter he became furious. He sent the following memo to Dr. English by registered mail:

> Either (1) you openly support the present structure of the clinic, including its style of supervision and its prescription writing policies, and be prepared to find ways to deal with legal and bureaucratic issues, *should* they arise; or (2) you accept the consequences of a legal and bureaucratic conservatism, which posits physician-centered health care delivery as a proper policy. The consequences of that approach are:
>
> 1. Fewer patients evaluated.
> 2. Fewer patients given follow-up care.
> 3. Greater costs per patient.

4. Fewer patients screened for important research.
5. Equating of a university mental health center to every other mental health center, no matter how mediocre, and equating of University Hospital's quality of care with that of every private psychiatrist, no matter how meretricious.

The department chairman was surprised by the memo since he had expected unquestioned compliance. He again was unsure how to proceed and was reluctant to go to Dr. Fineman for help. He decided to let the matter rest for a while.

* * * * *

Several weeks later, Dr. English met with the attorney and Ms. Liz Carey, the patients' rights coordinator for the hospital, to discuss a variety of patient-related issues. Ms. Carey mentioned a recent complaint referred to her from one of the patients in Dr. Rosen's clinic. The patient apparently was a medical school dropout who had been receiving care for several months. His complaint was that he had yet to see a physician and it appeared to him that the nurse was prescribing all of the medications for him. The patient was anxious to receive a response to his complaint.

Dr. English immediately tried to reach Dr. Rosen to discuss the matter. However, the latter was not in his office so Dr. English asked the patient's nurse clinician to come to his office. She explained that since she was a newcomer to the clinic she had discussed her assessment of the patient in great depth and on several occasions with Dr. Rosen. She said it was he who wrote prescriptions for the patient. Dr. English thanked her for the information and she left. The department chairman continued the discussion with Stoner and Ms. Carey.

About 15 minutes later, Dr. Rosen came storming into Dr. English's office. In the presence of Ms. Carey, Stoner, and Dr. English's secretary, Dr. Rosen shouted, "Lyle, what right do you have to go around me by talking to one of my nurses about an issue that should have been discussed solely with me! Don't you ever talk to anyone else in my clinic, patient or staff, without first clearing it with me."

Dr. English was embarrassed and tried to reason with Dr. Rosen. "Look," he said, "I didn't go around you. I tried to reach you first but you were out. I needed a quick answer on a matter requiring an immediate response."

Dr. Rosen abruptly turned and walked out, saying, "Don't let it happen again!"

A few days later, Dr. English received a typewritten letter from Dr. Rosen accompanied by the partially burned fragments of the registered letter of directions from the chairman. In the letter, Dr. Rosen criticized Dr. English for his poor leadership qualities which, he wrote, was a general view throughout the medical school and the hospital. Dr. Rosen wrote that, "My associates and I conclude that you couldn't lead a horse to water!" He also expressed the opinion that Dr. English was a better "public relations type" than anything else.

About the same time as the letter was received, two other events occurred. Dr. English heard a rumor that during a clinic office party Dr. Rosen was walking around with a wine bottle in his hand, challenging "Lyle" to face him "man to man." Dr. English also was requested by a nurse to provide care personally to a former patient of Dr. Rosen's clinic whom the latter had refused to see because of what he had termed the "patient's uncooperative and criminally dangerous nature."

* * * * *

Upset and frustrated over the whole matter, Dr. English made an appointment to see Dr. Fineman. At the meeting, the medical director pledged his support for any decision the department chairman recommended and suggested that Dr. English also might want to discuss the matter with Stoner, the hospital attorney.

Following that suggestion, Dr. English again met with Stoner, who already was familiar with many of the circumstances because of his previous opinion and his witnessing of the blow-up after Dr. English had talked with the nurse from Dr. Rosen's clinic. Stoner debated in his mind whether to give a written opinion to Dr. English. He decided against it because he felt that such a formality might limit the options open to the chairman. Instead he told Dr. English that the problem was complicated by Dr. Rosen's multiple job responsibilities and by the affiliation agreement between the hospital and the university. Therefore, the attorney based his discussion on Dr. Rosen's major roles and the policies applicable to each of them. He covered the following points:

- Dr. Rosen held a faculty appointment at the university, which was governed by university policies and procedures. These policies and procedures provided that appointments and promotions should, among other factors, consider a faculty member's capacity for cooperation with associates. The documents were not specific as to what kinds of actions by a faculty member were grounds for immediate discharge from employment and were silent on medical practice. It would reasonably be assumed, though, that administrative insubordination, defamation, and slander were sufficient grounds for dismissal. All faculty members obviously were entitled to initiate the university grievance process to air areas of disagreement with decisions that affected them.

- Dr. Rosen, as a member of the medical staff of University Hospital, was obliged to comply with the constitution and bylaws of the medical staff.

The bylaws provided that suspension of clinical privileges or revocation of staff membership could be initiated by the medical director or the president of the medical staff whenever "the activities or professional conduct of any individual are considered to be lower than, or in violation of, the standards of the hospital, or to be disruptive to the operations of hospital." The medical director or president of the medical staff could implement a summary suspension, effective immediately, whenever "because of immediate danger to a patient, action must be taken in the best interest of patient care in the hospital." Medical staff membership depended on annual reappointment, which was based on several factors, including a physician's ethics and conduct, cooperation with hospital personnel, and relations with other practitioners. Whenever a decision adversely affected medical staff membership, the affected person had the right to invoke due process review in the medical staff bylaws.

- Dr. Rosen, as the administrative head of a hospital clinic, was expected to comply with the rules and regulations of the hospital even though he was technically not a hospital employee. All hospital personnel were expected to cooperate with one another in a professional manner and to conform with all state and federal laws when performing their duties. As in the case of university faculty members and hospital medical staff members, hospital personnel also had the right to grieve, through a formal process, actions affecting them with which they disagreed.

Stoner advised Dr. English that, whatever action he decided to take, e.g., university, medical staff, hospital, or a combination of more than one, he also would have to consider the terms of the affiliation agreement between the university and the hospital. Stoner said it might not be possible to concentrate on any one area of Dr. Rosen's responsibilities without also involving serious consideration of the impact on all of the others.

Stoner voiced the opinion that Dr. Rosen appeared inappropriate in his personal relationships with Dr. English. The attorney also was concerned that the way in which Dr. Rosen had structured his clinic appeared to violate laws and regulations pertaining specifically to the prescription of drugs and, generally, to the practice of medicine. He made his concerns clear to Dr. English, warning that whatever action was taken, it must not appear that the sole reason for the action was a personality conflict between the two. The attorney then asked Dr. English what he hoped to accomplish in taking disciplinary action against Dr. Rosen.

The department chairman appeared overwhelmed and upset, in that so much of his time was being consumed by a problem that no one else would solve for him. His agitation was apparent in his response to Stoner.

"No one should treat anyone the way Dr. Rosen has treated me. Dr. Rosen has disregarded everything I have ever said to him, and he has taken it completely out of context. I don't think he is as good a clinician as he thinks he is. He is a damn buffoon, if you ask me! He is out to make me look a fool, too."

While listening, it became apparent to Stoner that Dr. Rosen's behavior was more important to Dr. English than the way in which he ran his clinic. Dr. English continued:

"You know, Jim, Dr. Fineman says he will support whatever decision I make. But you and I know that Dr. Rosen is his boy. Whatever I decide to do, I must respect how Dr. Fineman feels about Dr. Rosen's value to the university and the department. I guess I should be satisfied if Dr. Rosen apologizes to me for his behavior and knocks off some of those illegal practices in his clinic."

* * * * *

With that Dr. English asked Stoner to set up another meeting with Dr. Fineman to discuss a plan to deal with the clinic director. At that meeting they agreed that Dr. Fineman, Dr. English, and the hospital administrator, Franklin Hummer, should meet with Dr. Rosen, reprimand him for his conduct, and give him a choice of two alternatives:

1. He could apologize to Dr. English for his inappropriate conduct and accept a two-year probationary period. If he completed the probationary period without similar incident, the letter of reprimand would be withdrawn from his personnel file. Should he exhibit similar misconduct during that probation, he would be relieved of his administrative position as clinic director, and the special compensation associated with this position would be terminated.
2. He would be relieved of his position as clinic director along with its special compensation should he choose not to apologize, and in timely fashion.

Stoner was disappointed that there was so little discussion on the issue of how the clinic was run.

The meeting was held as agreed. Dr. Fineman as medical director opened by expressing his concerns over the seriousness of the matter. "Alan," he said to Dr. Rosen, "I think you know why you are here. I don't get involved in minor problems. This is important."

Dr. Rosen then was given an opportunity to respond to the allegations of misconduct against him as presented by Dr. Fineman. After listening quietly, he thought to himself that his real loyalty was to Dr. Fineman. He decided he could help the medical director out of his jam of trying to show support to Dr. English by being cooperative. When Dr. Fineman was finished, Dr. Rosen looked at Dr. English and said, "Lyle, I apologize. It won't happen again."

Dr. English was shocked and speechless. Hummer, the hospital adminstrator, was puzzled as to why physicians made such big things over such small issues. The meeting was adjourned by Dr. Fineman, who thanked all for their attendance and spirit of cooperation.

A few weeks later, Dr. Rosen was promoted to associate professor with tenure. In fact, the president of the medical staff, who appeared to know nothing about the incident with Dr. English, congratulated Dr. Rosen on his promotion and told him to keep up the good work.

To celebrate his promotion, Dr. Rosen purchased his first Cadillac. He wasn't even 40 yet. Well, he thought, he would buy a Mercedes when he was promoted to full professor.

Commentary

1.

Cost effectiveness and maximizing reimbursement are primary concerns in the delivery of health care services. The use of nonphysicians such as nurse practitioners and physician assistants is one possible answer to these problems. However, laws and regulations on the practice of medicine, as well as reimbursement rules, are unclear and apparently conservative about how nonphysicians may be used independent of, or ancillary to, physicians in patient care.

This is a particularly difficult problem in psychiatry, where there is considerable overlap in what physicians, nurses, social workers, psychologists, and other mental health professionals do for patients. It is not unusual for physicians (and hospital administrators) to be misled by policies and pressures that are not consistent with laws and regulations.

The irony is that cost containment has an impact across the board on the delivery of health care services, including medical practice, e.g., number of tests, amount of surgery, etc., yet the use of nonphysicians to lower costs may not be reimbursable from a third party payer standpoint.

2.

The multiple roles and goals that exist in academic health centers can make coping with faculty personnel issues a most difficult process. In the Rosen case, it appears that hospital and university officials were in agreement. But suppose they were not? What would have happened if Dr. Rosen had lost faculty privileges but had retained hospital privileges, or the reverse? Does the university have an obligation to assure clinical privileges for its faculty members who are physicians? Who has primary responsibility for clinical directors—the hospital administration, the university administration, or the hospital medical staff? Hospitals and universities must be careful about what they promise their physicians about clinical practice and academic rank.

3.

Physicians, like everyone else, do not always get along with their superiors. The medical profession and the academic community have always had an aversion to such concepts as hierarchy, chain of command, and direct supervision. However, the courts are increasingly recognizing that the disciplining of a physician is justified where inability to work with others affects patient care. Some views of professional independence and academic freedom are likely to clash with institutional needs and prerogatives.

4.

Hospital, university, and medical staff members all expose themselves to liability risk when it is known, or even suspected, that a hospital clinic may be providing patient care in a manner contrary to law or regulation. The fact that the quality of care generally is considered good is not a defense from a legal standpoint since litigation usually is the result of a bad outcome. Furthermore, courts ordinarily wait for legislators to change the law and are not sympathetic toward physicians and hospital administrators who go off on their own.

In that connection, institutions have the responsibility to prevent persons from practicing medicine who are not legally qualified to do so; they run the risk of being subject to penalties for aiding and abetting illegal practice.

5.

In the case study, Dr. Rosen was not given specific details about the meeting he was to have with Dr. Fineman, Dr. English, and Hummer, the hospital administrator, concerning his conduct. Nor was he advised as to whether or not he had the right to bring legal representation or witnesses. Quite often persons who are to be disciplined are not formally advised about their rights prior to the meetings that discuss their conduct.

The question as to how formal such preliminary meetings should be is important. Formality has a tendency to reduce flexibility and to eliminate options that might well have been satisfactory to all parties concerned had it not been for the rigid process. An informal process may make it possible to prevent the escalation of a matter to one that will require a long and costly formal adjudication.

It is possible that the presence of Stoner, the house counsel for the hospital, at the final meeting with Dr. Rosen may have added more formality to the process than was necessary and, if the session had not concluded as it did, would have supported a complaint by Dr. Rosen that he was not given an opportunity for representation and thus was denied due process during the discussions.

6.

Dr. Rosen's academic appointment also raises some important considerations. In most academic health settings there are two kinds of faculty—private practitioners who are clinical faculty, and full-time academic clinical faculty. The power base usually resides with the latter with respect to the research, teaching, and services provided in the hospital.

This, of course, creates conflict between the two types of faculty and minimizes the role that the private practitioner member can play in many situations, particularly those involving the full-time academic clinical faculty. It also is unclear as to the extent to which the clinical practice and conduct of full-time academic clinical faculty members should affect their promotion within the academic setting. Popularity and the cooperative spirit are not necessary prerequisites for academic achievement in research.

7.

It appears that none of the individuals in the case study were concerned about discussing the situation with the hospital medical staff. In this respect the case demonstrates the rather low priority and importance of the traditional medical staff organization that exists in many academic health centers. The president of the medical staff of University Hospital never was involved in the Rosen situation, a matter relating to patient care and professional conduct with which the medical staff of a community hospital almost always is deeply involved.

8.

Finally, the case demonstrates some of the difficulties hospital house counsel may experience. Counsel must be objective and recognize the variety of interests that must be balanced in reaching recommendations. Part of the house counsel's problem is in determining who the client is when a particular problem is presented.

Counsel must keep in mind to whom particular advice is given and how it will be used. Requests often are made to house counsel for advice to support one faction of the hospital community against another. Regardless of how careful the attorney is, the net effect may be that the individual may end up in the middle of a conflict because the lawyer's professional opinion may favor one position at the expense of another.

Case 8

Facing Up

PERSONAE

Dr. B.J. Adler, member of hearing panel

Dr. Frank Blair, emergency room physician, East Side General Hospital

Dr. James Buchanan, president of Hope medical staff and chairman of Medical Staff Executive Committee

Dr. Louis Capolla, member of hearing panel

William Connors, administrator of East Side General

Dr. Howard Cook, member of hearing panel

Dr. Seymour Cooper, endocrinologist, East Side General Hospital, treating physician for Dr. Morgan

Paul Desberg, chairman of Hope Board of Trustees

Dr. Stephanie Fleming, member of hearing panel

David Gormon, Hope director of pharmacy

Linda Holmes, Hope nurse who moonlighted at East Side General

Dr. Stuart Levy, Hope physician criticized by Dr. Morgan

Peter Martin, Dr. Morgan's attorney

Dr. John Morgan, on staff of Hope Memorial Hospital, protagonist

Dr. Nathan Post, staff physician, Hope Memorial Hospital

Joan Ruud, nurse at Hope Memorial

Dr. Mark Sanders, physician who examined Dr. Morgan

Gordon Scott, attorney for Hope Memorial Hospital

Janet Starr, emergency room nurse, East Side General

Sara Stilton, nurse at Hope Memorial Hospital
Dr. Ralph Thomas, chief of medicine at Hope Memorial Hospital
Dr. Phillip Warner, internist, chairman of ad hoc hearing committee
George White, administrator of Hope Memorial Hospital

Saturday, July 25, 1981

A small crowd was gathered in the parking lot of King's Liquor Store. As Dr. Nathan Post approached, he saw a middle-aged man lying on the pavement, seemingly unconscious. He ascertained from a bystander that the man had suddenly fallen and was having some kind of seizure, and that an ambulance already had been called. Dr. Post identified himself as a physician and quickly began to examine the prone man, noting the alarmingly weak pulse, cold, clammy skin, and muscle flaccidity. He also noticed what appeared to to be multiple injection sites on the man's arms.

He asked a bystander to look in the stricken man's wallet for information and learned that the person was Dr. John Morgan, a physician on the staff at Hope Memorial Hospital. The bystander also noted a Diabetic Alert card in the wallet, which he showed to Dr. Post. When the ambulance arrived at the lot, the chief EMT took charge and said he was taking the patient to East Side General Hospital, the nearest hospital with emergency room facilities. Dr. Post followed in his own car, completely forgetting to buy the wine he had set out to purchase.

In the Emergency Room, Dr. Post reported the events at the parking lot, Dr. Morgan's symptoms, and his probable diabetic condition to Dr. Frank Blair, the physician on duty, who immediately began to evaluate the patient for the cause of the observed seizure and comatose state. He ordered a laboratory work-up, including blood sugar, acetone, electrolytes, and toxicology; arterial blood gas; and an EKG. He started therapy immediately, including intravenous dextrose.

Meanwhile, Janet Starr, the nurse on duty, looked through the papers in Dr. Morgan's wallet, hoping to find the name of his next of kin and any medically relevant information. In addition to the Diabetic Alert card, she found a business card from Dr. Seymour Cooper, an endocrinologist on East Side General's staff, which she showed to Dr. Blair.

"Good work, Janet," he grinned, "I hope Morgan is his patient. Page Dr. Cooper for me, will you? I'm pretty sure he's in the hospital."

Dr. Cooper was making rounds when he answered the page. Dr. Blair said, "A Dr. John Morgan has just been brought into emergency with possible insulin shock, Seymour. Is he your patient, by any chance? We found your card in his wallet."

"Why, yes, John Morgan has been my patient for several years," Dr. Cooper replied. "I just saw him two weeks ago and everything checked out then, but his condition has been quite serious. I'll be right down."

When Dr. Cooper arrived in the Emergency Room, Dr. Post was still there and described the patient's collapse. Dr. Morgan's condition had stabilized by that time, although he remained unconscious. The lab test indicated his blood sugar levels were low, suggesting that he was suffering from insulin shock. The tests did not show any other abnormal findings. Dr. Cooper took over from Dr. Blair, ordered the standard treatment for insulin shock and admission of his patient to the Intensive Care Unit.

Dr. Post saw no reason to remain any longer, commenting, "Looks like everything is under control here. First time I've ever been a Good Samaritan for another doctor. This will be tough on his patients."

As he was on his way to his car, he muttered, "Damn, now I won't have time to get that sauvignon blanc for George White's party."

* * * * *

Nurse Linda Holmes, who was regularly employed as a staff nurse at Hope Memorial Hospital, was moonlighting that weekend at East Side General, where she had been assigned to the Intensive Care Unit. She had a reputation as an extremely conscientious individual who believed not only in providing patients with top-quality nursing care but also in complying with any and all hospital rules and regulations. Fellow workers often described her as rigid and compulsive.

Upon Dr. Morgan's admission to the Intensive Care Unit, Nurse Holmes reviewed his chart and immediately realized that this was the very same John Morgan who was on the staff at Hope Memorial. She was aware of rumors among the nurses at Hope Memorial that something was seriously wrong with Dr. Morgan. He appeared to be under a great deal of stress and was having difficulties getting along with attending physicians as well as with the nursing staff.

She searched her memory for the recent conversation she heard among the other nurses.

"Ah, I know," she mused. "It was that big-mouthed Sara Stilton in the cafeteria last week. She said she overheard Dr. Morgan arguing with another doctor over some treatment, right in front of his patient, and loud, too. She exaggerates an awful lot, though. You'd think there was enough excitement in our line of work without her mouth adding to it.

"Hmmm, I remember Joan Ruud said something, too, and she's not usually one to pass on silly talk. She's a fine nurse, in the old style. Didn't she tell me that Dr. Morgan wouldn't let her give his patients their shots? That's right, she said he insisted on personally administering Demerol to two patients who were in severe pain. Neither one got any relief from his injections, either. She said she couldn't reach him for hours afterward. He just didn't answer the calls . . . And then, wasn't I there when he challenged Dr. Stuart Levy's judgment, causing that stupid scene in front of all those nurses and patients? Maybe that's the story that big-mouth Stilton was passing on."

* * * * *

Dr. Post arrived nearly two hours late for George White's cocktail party that evening and the Whites greeted him warmly. White was the administrator at Hope Memorial. Dr. Post, who recently joined the staff, was eager to attend and to meet some of the other administrators and staff physicans.

"I must apologize for arriving late and for failing to bring you the bottle of sauvignon blanc I promised you," Dr. Post said. "On my way to King's to buy the wine, I found myself in the role of Good Samaritan and I went on over to East Side General with a man who'd collapsed in the parking lot. Sort of a strange episode, really. The man was Dr. Morgan. You'd think an M.D. would be particularly careful and aware if he was diabetic. As a matter of fact, the fellow is on the staff here at Hope, although I haven't met him yet."

White was surprised and concerned. He said, "Dr. Morgan is one of ours. Some of his patients could be needing him."

"Well, George, when I left he was in good hands," Dr. Post said. "He was going up to the Intensive Care Unit. A Dr. Seymour Cooper was with him—said he'd been taking care of him for years. As a matter of fact, the worst worry you might have here is that Dr. Morgan might have been going to King's to buy you some wine, too! Everyone knows what an oenophile you are. I'm afraid you lost two good bottles on the same night."

Although he smiled at Dr. Post's last comment, White was a bit worried. He excused himself to call the admitting office. Unfortunately, the office confirmed what he had hoped would not be the case: Dr. Morgan had three patients in the hospital. He called the various nurses' stations to see whether Dr. Morgan had made rounds that day or, if not, whether any other physician had seen these patients on his behalf. None had. He called Dr. Morgan's office and got the answering service; then tried his home, again receiving no response. White assumed no arrangements had been made for the care of Dr. Morgan's patients so he called Hope's chief of medicine, Dr. Ralph Thomas, and briefly explained the circumstances surrounding the events of the last few hours.

"I thought something was going on with him," Dr. Thomas said. "I know he is a diabetic and has had some problems in controlling the disease, but I think he is being treated by that hotshot endocrinologist, Seymour Cooper, who's over at East Side General. Of course, Morgan's son's suicide last year has not helped matters. I don't know who usually covers for John. He's been quite a loner since his divorce, you know, but let me check it out and make sure that his patients in the hospital are seen and that his practice is covered for emergencies.

Dr. Thomas hesitated, then said,"There's something else about Dr. Morgan that I'd better tell you."

"I've heard quite enough for today," White responded. "If it is important, we could get together tomorrow, though."

"I think you ought to hear this, Mr. White," Dr. Thomas replied gravely. "Let's meet for breakfast. Is 11 o'clock good for you?"

* * * * *

Sunday, July 26,1981

Dr. Thomas, the Hope Memorial chief of medicine, and White, the hospital administrator, met, as arranged, in a small, elegant restaurant on the outskirts of Packersburg. After he ordered his eggs Benedict, White urged Dr. Thomas to get right to business. Dr. Thomas laid out the situation:

"John Morgan is 45 years old. He's been on the staff at Hope Memorial Hospital for the last 16 years. By the standards of the medical profession, he has everything going for him. He graduated at the top of his class from Johns Hopkins and trained in Boston. In the past he has been meticulous in his practice, has carried a heavy workload, and has been demanding of himself and associates.

"Everything seemed to be going fairly well for him until his divorce about three years ago and the suicide of his 17-year-old son last year. No one knows why his son killed himself and John has been strongly affected by it. He seemed to feel personally responsible for allowing his former wife to have custody of the boy and for failing to perceive early indications of his unhappiness.

"Changes in Morgan's behavior and activities appeared subtly at first. He began to miss conferences and meetings at the hospital. His office practice, which had been well organized, began to fall into disarray. Then complaints from colleagues, nurses, and patients began to surface. Patients said he would not fill out insurance forms and would not send their records to other physicians when they asked him to do so. They also complained that he failed to keep appointments with them.

"In addition, several doctors in the department complained to me that his medical decisions and judgments often were flawed, his pattern of patient rounds had become erratic and unpredictable, and his hospital chart entries were interminably long and illegible. Some nurses mentioned his increasingly rude behavior and told me that it had become very difficult to work with him.

"At first, I gave these complaints little attention. I was well aware of Dr. Morgan's personal situation and felt sure that his professional problems were only temporary. I believed that John merely needed some time to work out his personal difficulties. In view of his long and successful association with Hope, I wanted to give him a second chance."

White thought privately that it didn't sound too bad so far. He leaned forward and said, "I'm sure you did the right thing then, Ralph. But I'm also certain you wouldn't be here with me now if it had stopped there."

"Unfortunately, you're right," the chief of medicine replied. With a sigh, he continued:

"About three months ago I decided that the time had come to thoroughly investigate the complaints against Dr. Morgan. After all, as chief I have a responsibility to the hospital, its staff, and its patients to ensure that, to the best of my knowledge, the physicians on my service are meeting the highest standards of professional conduct and competence.

"Before I could decide on my next step, David Gormon, the director of the hospital pharmacy, came to see me. Gormon is intelligent, hard-working, and conscientious. I believe he has held his position for six years and is generally considered to have done a fine job. I respected Gormon's judgment, and what he told me was especially disturbing, given the high opinion I have of him.

"Gormon informed me that he believed he had recognized a potential drug problem in one of the physicians in the department. Over the past six months, it appeared that Dr. Morgan had ordered greater and greater quantities of Demerol, that these quantities now exceeded the average prescription orders of other physicians in my department, and that many of these orders did not appear to be medically necessary. Gormon said he had questioned Dr. Morgan on a few occasions concerning the orders and that Morgan had exploded in a rage, insisting that Gormon had better watch his step if he wanted to keep his job at Hope Memorial.

"Although Gormon said he was not certain that Dr. Morgan did, in fact, have a drug problem, or any other problem, he felt that I should know about the situation. I was absolutely shocked by the information, as I can see you are. I assured Dave that I would personally look into the matter and I asked him not to mention his suspicions to anyone else. He agreed to my request."

The hospital administrator stared grimly at his chief of medicine. His mouth had become a thin, whitened line and his left eyelid was twitching almost imperceptibly.

"Go on, Ralph," White said, "but let's get some more coffee to go with the rest of this story first."

Tension showed in Dr. Thomas's face, too, as he watched the waiter fill his cup. A vertical ridge of furrows had appeared between his widely spaced eyes and his tanned face took on a look of resignation. He went on.

"As soon as possible I met with Dr. Morgan and confronted him with all the complaints and allegations of professional misconduct that had been brought to my attention. I stressed that the purpose of our meeting was not accusatory in nature. Rather, I told him, I wanted to hear his side of the story and to correct any potential problems before they got out of hand.

"He vehemently denied the existence of any drug-related problem and said it should be obvious to me that some troublemakers at the hospital were out to get him and were trying to jeopardize his association with Hope. He explained that his absences from hospital and departmental meetings over the past several months were the result of his ex-wife's personal problems. It seems she had a nervous breakdown after their son's suicide, and although they were no longer married, he often felt bound to be with her, despite his other obligations.

"George, he argued his case quite well in some ways. He said his practice still was flourishing and that he was having no trouble seeing patients when he was really needed. He also said that his 16 years in practice and his intelligence combined to enable him to teach nearly every topic at the departmental meetings. He told me he was up on all the new techniques in the field and he resented me and the rest of the staff looking over his shoulder all the time.

"Then it was my turn. I stressed to Dr. Morgan that I was aware of the strain his son's suicide had placed on him and his ex-wife. I added that I felt that he had failed to challenge two important allegations: the report that he had been submitting excessive prescriptions for Demerol to the hospital pharmacy and the complaints from physicians, nurses, and patients regarding his professional behavior or, rather, his unprofessional behavior.

"I told him that I expected him to make regular patient rounds, to record accurate physician notes in patient charts, to make every effort to get along with the nursing staff, and to attend department meetings and conferences. Moreover, I said that I would personally review the quantities and types of narcotics he ordered from the hospital pharmacy, and that excessive prescriptions of Demerol or any other drug must not occur.

"George, I did reaffirm my confidence in his past professionalism and I suggested that he seek appropriate help to get him through this very difficult period if he needed it. I also promised him that our meeting and its contents would remain confidential."

At this point, White's hand trembled, causing him to spill a little of his coffee. His face had tightened further, though all he said was, "Go on, Ralph, I must hear the entire story."

"Well, John adamantly restated his position," Dr. Thomas continued. "He said he was not guilty of professional misconduct or incompetence, that the complaints raised in no way indicated or reflected any drug abuse on his part, and that he was shocked that, after 16 years of impeccable service to Hope Memorial and this community, the troublemaker, whose identity he refused to reveal, had been able to persuade me to turn against him. He did agree to cooperate with me fully to resolve the matter and we decided to meet periodically to discuss his progress.

"However, since that meeting, Dr. Morgan's professional conduct has improved only minimally. Although he has attended scheduled meetings, he has continued to make patient rounds at odd hours, and his medical chart entries are even more sloppy and inconcise than they were. In addition, his orders for Demerol continue to be far above the department average.

"Frankly, George, I would not be at all surprised if Dr. Morgan's seizure in the parking lot were connected with all this in some way."

White had been the administrator at Hope Memorial for just two years. Never before had he been faced with a situation involving a possible drug-abusing physician and he did not know the exact procedures the hospital should follow. He was furious that Dr. Thomas had not informed him of the situation until this day. He thought to himself, "Dr. Morgan has been a threat not only to himself but to his patients and the hospital as well." He felt that Dr. Thomas had kept the matter private for too long, although he said nothing of his thoughts. He did say with taut restraint:

"A physician shouldn't have to overdose in a public place before anything is brought to my attention. I'm sorely disappointed in you, Ralph. My first priority, as yours should be, is the quality of patient care at Hope. Please make the necessary arrangements for Dr. Morgan's patients in the house to be assigned to other staff physicians."

Dr. Thomas stood abruptly and said, "That has already been taken care of, George. Is there anything else you want me to do? If not, I must be going."

He walked stiffly to his car, cheeks burning with anger, and sat hunched over the wheel for several minutes before he finally straightened his shoulders, stabbed his key into the ignition, and drove home, exceeding the speed limit most of the way. He consoled himself with the thought that any physician would have tried to help a fellow doctor the way he had.

"Well, what can you expect from an administrator," he thought. "He's just a lay person, after all." Still, it rankled that White did not appreciate his efforts to solve the problem quickly and save the medical profession and the hospital from embarrassment. At the time he failed to appreciate that White was worrying about just that issue—the serious blot on the hospital's reputation if the story came out.

* * * * *

White had remained at the table in the restaurant. He ordered a brandy and began to think rapidly, methodically, about the serious, long-term problem he had on his hands. He had worked hard to get where he was. Hope Memorial had an excellent reputation in the state—a reputation he had helped to build. Located in Packersburg, a stable eastern city with a population of half a million, Hope competed for patients and staff with several other large hospitals. He had not gotten this far only to have his reputation tarnished.

In his upward climb he had worked hard to ensure that the top job in such a fine hospital would come his way. He smugly recalled negotiating the terrific financial deal he had made before accepting the post, and began to picture the paneled walnut conference room where he has sat with the president of the board—which now was his conference room . . .

Forcibly, he pulled himself away from his reverie and decided that what he needed was more information about John Morgan's present illness and condition. Typical, that all this aggravation over a doctor should happen on a weekend.

* * * * *

Meanwhile, Nurse Linda Holmes's curiosity as to the cause of Dr. Morgan's illness was aroused even further than it had been initially when his condition failed to improve under standard insulin shock therapy. When she came on duty at East Side General at 3 P.M. Sunday, she decided to focus on him. She learned he had regained consciousness and had become unruly, with periods of disorientation and confusion as well as seizure-like activity. Yet repeat blood analyses revealed no systemic dysfunction. Nurse Holmes's suspicions were confirmed by a note Dr. Cooper had entered in Dr. Morgan's chart earlier that day that the initial seizure and current aberrant behavior might be related to an underlying metabolic abnormality, or alcohol or drug withdrawal state.

She was extremely disturbed upon reading Dr. Cooper's note. She recently had attended a conference sponsored by the local county nursing association at which one of the major discussion topics was the new state statute requiring hospital administrators, physicians, and nurses to report all instances of professional misconduct to the State Board of Medical Examiners. Nurse Holmes recalled that professional misconduct included practicing one's profession while impaired by alcohol or drugs. She resolved to seek the advice of the director of nursing at Hope Memorial first thing Monday morning.

* * * * *

Monday, July 27, 1981

White's first item of business that morning was to telephone his counterpart, William Connors, the administrator at East Side General Hospital. The two men had met at several social occasions in the last two years so he felt comfortable asking Connors for confirmation of Dr. Morgan's admission and even for further information about his condition. After checking, Connors replied:

"Yes, George, your Dr. Morgan was admitted over the weekend and he is still in the Intensive Care Unit. I really shouldn't say any more about the case, technically, but listen George, you've got a real problem on your hands. I'm telling you this because if one of my doctors is ever in your hospital, I hope you'll do the same for me. Dr. Morgan appears to be going through some kind of withdrawal right now. I'm no doctor, so I don't know if this means he's addicted to something or what. All I know is that he'll probably be well enough to leave here soon and I hope you're prepared for his return. And remember, you didn't hear any of this from me."

White thanked Connors solemnly and hung up, with a sinking feeling about the serious situation that had erupted. He telephoned Dr. Morgan's treating physician, Dr. Cooper. He explained his position at Hope Memorial and his concern for Dr. Morgan's practice and patients. He added, "I understand that Dr. Morgan is still in the ICU and is unable to have visitors. Can you provide me with an update on his condition?"

Dr. Cooper replied, "Dr. Morgan is in stable condition and although I'd like to be able to tell you more, I really can't. As his physician, I need his okay before I talk to you. You'll have to ask him about his condition when he is able to have visitors. I'm sure you know that Dr. Morgan could sue me if I disclose anything about his situation."

White was not surprised by Dr. Cooper's response. He knew how suit-conscious many doctors were, although he wondered if the confidentiality ethic should be bent when the patient was a so-called "impaired physician." Dr. Morgan's current hospitalization and the possibility of his drug addiction convinced White that some action had to be taken to suspend his hospital privileges temporarily until a complete investigation could be made.

The problem was, however, that the hospital's medical staff bylaws provided only for a summary suspension or a voluntary medical leave of absence, and neither procedure was technically correct in this instance. In this case, Dr. Morgan had not purposely abandoned his patients; he had fallen ill, seemingly without any forewarning. It would be unfair and arbitrary to suspend his privileges without a clear finding of wrongdoing. A summary suspension usually was reserved for situations that created an immediate threat to patient health and safety, or intentional physician misconduct or neglect.

Although the alternative of a medical leave of absence would have been a good solution, in that the hospital would have been afforded the opportunity to review Dr. Morgan before his return to practice from the leave, the bylaws provided that a request for a medical leave of absence must be made by the physician concerned. Clearly, at this time, Dr. Morgan was physically incapable of making such a request, even if he would agree to do so.

As White sat, toying with these options in his mind, his secretary said Nurse Linda Holmes was in the outer office and she was asking to see him immediately regarding an urgent matter. White asked that she be shown in. Nurse Holmes came right to the point.

"Mr. White, the director of nursing felt I should see you directly about this problem. You see, I was moonlighting over at East Side General this weekend when a physician on our staff was brought in to the ICU. We thought he had collapsed from insulin shock, but he really wasn't responding to treatment. I saw a note on his chart from Dr. Cooper, his attending physician, which is why I'm here. The note indicated that he might be going through a drug withdrawal reaction."

White shifted uncomfortably in his chair, looked down at his carefully manicured, elegantly slender hands, and said, "That must have been upsetting for you, Miss Holmes."

"Well, yes. It is upsetting and it puts me in a predicament. During the last meeting of the nurses' association, the speaker was a lawyer who said we are required by a law to report any incident that showed that a doctor might be impaired. Do you think this is a case of physician impairment of the kind he was talking about? I've been worrying about it ever since I saw that note on the chart."

White cautiously acknowledged that he understood the import of her question. "Miss Holmes, I'm not really sure of the answer to your question," he hedged. "I'm quite concerned about it, too, and I think the hospital is obligated to find the right answer under the circumstances."

Inwardly, White thanked her for her tact in not referring to Dr. Morgan by name. He wondered how many others knew already what Nurse Holmes knew, and what they might be planning to do about it. He said:

"I appreciate your coming to me with this problem before you reported it to the State Board of Medical Examiners. What I'd like to do is check into the matter very carefully and then let you know what I've learned. Will you please wait until I can get back to you?"

Nurse Holmes was a bit relieved to acquiesce. She felt a little sorry for Dr. Morgan even though he had been acting pretty oddly. She said, as she rose to leave, "I'll be glad to hold off for a little while, just as long as I know I can do what's right in the long run."

* * * * *

As soon as she left, White decided it was incumbent upon the hospital to impose a forced medical leave of absence on Dr. Morgan, despite the lack of such a procedure in the medical staff bylaws. He reasoned that when a staff physician was hospitalized, an immediate medical leave of absence from the medical staff was called for.

Although White was convinced that the evidence he had gathered thus far indicated that Dr. Morgan in fact had a drug problem, he felt there would be many difficulties in getting hard evidence if corrective action were sought against him later.

Bill Connors, the East Side General administrator, clearly would refuse to testify; besides, his evidence was third hand. Dr. Cooper would be unlikely to testify because of his view of the physician-patient relationship and, in addition, White was aware of federal regulations concerning the confidentiality of alcohol and drug abuse patient records. He made a mental note to check further to see whether those regulations might affect the hospital's ability to get documentation and information about Dr. Morgan's condition.

White arranged for Dr. Thomas, the chief of medicine, and Dr. James Buchanan, president of the medical staff and chairman of the Medical Staff Executive Committee, to meet with him in his office late in the day. After he explained the situation to Dr. Buchanan and brought Dr. Thomas up to date, he said, "I think it is advisable to impose a forced medical leave of absence on Dr. Morgan. Since the bylaws provide only for the grant of a voluntary leave of medical absence, I will have to write a new procedure to cover this situation."

Dr. Buchanan responded, "The Medical Staff Executive Committee won't be meeting until late next month, so if you insist on taking immediate action, you will have to do so without ratification by us."

"I know, I know," White answered impatiently. "I am determined to proceed without delay. Clearly, the committee can ratify the hospital's position at its next meeting. A procedural technicality should not preclude the hospital from taking necessary and appropriate action. As I see it, when a staff physician becomes ill and can't carry on his practice, the chief of that physician's department, the president of the medical staff, and the administrator of the hospital may decide, together, to grant an immediate and temporary medical leave of absence without the request or consent of the affected doctor. I concede that our action should be subject to ratification by the executive committee at its next session, of course."

Faced with the urgency of the situation and the recognition that Dr. Morgan had patients in the hospital, the three agreed to act immediately.

White said, "I'll let you both know when the necessary documents are ready for your signatures," and Dr. Thomas agreed to call Dr. Morgan's office to let his secretary know how his hospitalized patients were to be handled and help the person make referrals for his office practice. Dr. Morgan had had no associate in his office for more than three years and generally made ad hoc coverage arrangements as best he could.

* * * * *

Tuesday, July 28, 1981

By the next afternoon, White had prepared a memorandum to be submitted to the Medical Staff Executive Committee concerning the temporary leave of absence imposed on Dr. Morgan and the reasons therefor. In the memorandum he suggested that this procedure be formalized and incorporated into the bylaws for similar future situations. White then prepared a letter to Dr. Morgan that he and Drs. Buchanan and Thomas signed, stating that he had been granted a medical leave of absence effective immediately. The letter was sent to Dr. Morgan's residence, with copies to his office and to the admitting and medical staff offices of the hospital.

* * * * *

Thursday, July 30, 1981

Dr. Morgan was discharged from East Side General the fifth day. When he arrived home he was shocked to find White's letter among the mail that had accumulated. Upon reading it, he exploded in a rage. The letter was as follows:

> July 28, 1981
> Dear Dr. Morgan,
> Because of your recent illness and hospitalization, we are granting you a temporary leave of absence from the Medical Staff, effective immediately. As a matter of policy, it is very important that we receive a complete report on your physical health from all the physicians who were vitally involved in your care so that we can make an appropriate recommendation concerning your leave of absence to the Medical Staff Executive Committee. Please have the appropriate physicians, therefore, send reports soon, so that we can act on your leave of absence, which is currently in force.
> Sincerely,
> /s/*George White,* Administrator
> Hope Memorial Hospital
> /s/*James Buchanan,* M.D.
> /s/*Ralph Thomas,* M.D.

Dr. Morgan immediately rushed to Hope Memorial. He stormed into the Department of Medicine office, where Dr. Thomas was reviewing some papers, shouting and waving the letter he had just received. Enraged, he sputtered, "You broke our agreement to maintain confidentiality! You promised to keep quiet about those complaints and our agreement. I kept my part of the bargain! Why didn't you?"

Still shouting, Dr. Morgan insisted that Dr. Thomas immediately lift the leave of absence.

The chief of medicine hardly expected the hospital's action to meet with Dr. Morgan's approval. He began to speak calmingly after Dr. Morgan had finished. He said he stood by the content of the letter:

"You suffered an unexplained illness that caused you to be hospitalized. You were unable to continue your practice during that illness and we cannot be sure that you are capable of resuming your practice at the hospital unless and until you submit a report from your treating physician stating that you are physically able to return to your work. Reinstatement will not be considered without that report."

Although Dr. Morgan argued strenuously, Dr. Thomas remained unmoved and Dr. Morgan stormed out.

* * * * *

Friday, July 31, 1981

Dr. Morgan knew he could not ask his treating physician for a statement on his physical condition because Dr. Cooper was noticeably suspicious about the cause of the recent episode. Dr. Morgan decided that it would be best to see a doctor who didn't know him or anything about him, so he made an appointment for the following Monday, with Dr. Mark Sanders, a young practitioner in a small city 25 miles away, for a complete physical examination. He had met Dr. Sanders at a social event a year or so previously and believed he knew few people at Hope Memorial.

* * * * *

Monday, August 3, 1981

Dr. Sanders examined and found Dr. Morgan to be generally in good health, with his diabetes apparently under control. Dr. Morgan said he needed a letter for an insurance company, stating that he had been examined by a physician and that he had been found to be in good physical health. Dr. Sanders said, "I'll be happy to write this letter for you. Why don't you leave the address of the insurance carrier with my secretary?"

Dr. Morgan said he didn't know the address offhand and asked Dr. Sanders to mail the letter to his home address.

* * * * *

Tuesday, August 4, 1981

Upon receipt of Dr. Sanders's letter, Dr. Morgan wasted no time in submitting it to Dr. Thomas, who was not satisfied.

"I need a letter from your regular treating physician," the chief of medicine declared. "Dr. Sanders indicates that he has examined you only on this one occasion. Moreover, his report doesn't even mention your recent hospitalization at East Side General.

"It's my understanding that for the past several years you have been under a Dr. Cooper's care for treatment of a diabetic condition and that Dr. Cooper was in charge of your case at East Side General. A letter from Dr. Cooper is what I need. I don't understand why you saw Dr. Sanders instead of Dr. Cooper."

Dr. Morgan was furious.

"I complied with your request," he raged. "I got you the letter. Now you claim it's not good enough. I believe I still have the right to choose my treating physician. Dr. Sanders is now my treating physician, not Dr. Cooper. Your unreasonable refusal to end the leave of absence is costing me my patients and my practice. If you and the hospital want a lawsuit on your hands, you'll have one!"

* * * * *

Later that day, Dr. Morgan telephoned Peter Martin, an attorney he had met three years earlier when he testified on behalf of one of his patients in a malpractice action against another physician who had treated the person previously. After briefly describing his problem, Dr. Morgan made an appointment for the following morning to discuss his legal options in light of Dr. Thomas's refusal to lift the medical leave of absence.

* * * * *

Wednesday, August 5, 1981

Dr. Morgan stomped into the attorney's office and threw himself into a chair, saying, "These bastards are hounding me! I can't take care of my patients because I'm not on their staff. This letter here, damn it, is causing me to lose income and my good name! They aren't going to get away with this!"

He waved the letter in front of the lawyer's face, then put it in Martin's hands.

"Well, now, Dr. Morgan, let's just see what we can do about this," soothed Martin, who'd experienced quite a few clients with ruffled feathers before. "Can you tell me some more about this letter and about the hospital's bylaws, especially with regard to appointments and leaves of absence?"

Required to think about such substantive issues, Dr. Morgan slowed down considerably, as Martin knew he would. He was forced to admit to the attorney he knew very little about those procedures and so, moving through that crack in his facade of rage and affronted dignity, Martin settled in to get the facts from John Morgan's point of view. They discussed in general Hope Memorial's history and its rules and procedures governing physicians' activities and staff privileges.

By the time they'd gotten through with all that, Dr. Morgan was able to go into his personal story more quietly.

"Eleven days ago, I was hospitalized at East Side General for my diabetic condition," he said. "It was nothing serious and I was released after a few days with a clean bill of health."

While he spoke, Dr. Morgan nervously twisted a heavy ring round and round on his finger. He obviously was trying to keep his voice under control but it shook as he went on:

"During my hospitalization, Dr. Thomas, my department chief, who was supposed to be my friend, instituted this forced medical leave of absence against me. He didn't even go to the Medical Staff Executive Committee for consent. I can't understand how he could be so hypocritical!

"I tried to comply with their conditions for reinstatement. I had a complete physical and gave Dr. Thomas a complete report. It says my diabetes is under control and that there is no reason why I should not resume my practice."

Dr. Morgan handed the lawyer a copy of Dr. Sanders's report, saying, "Dr. Thomas had the nerve to reject this report as inadequate. He insists on one from Seymour Cooper, who is no longer my treating physician."

Martin sat behind his enormous walnut desk, listening carefully and thinking that his client looked like his 4-year-old nephew when he was refused an extra piece of cake after dinner, with the exception of the shadow of his dark beard beneath the otherwise smooth, almost childlike features. The attorney pushed his heavy horn-rimmed spectacles back over his head and rubbed his eyes. Then he said:

"I can't properly advise you until I have had a chance to review the hospital and medical staff bylaws concerning corrective action and the imposition of a forced medical leave of absence, Dr. Morgan. Is there anything else you want to tell me about all this? Do you want to consider getting the report from Dr. Cooper, just to have this matter closed?"

Dr. Morgan looked a bit sheepish at that but quickly recovered his air of injured innocence.

"It's a matter of principle, now, Pete," he said. "I may call you Pete? Yes. I am not going to let them tell me whom I may choose as my personal physician and I'm not going to let Ralph Thomas keep me off that staff!"

Dr. Morgan agreed to get both sets of bylaws for his lawyer before their next meeting. As they shook hands, he said gruffly, "Thanks, I feel like I might get somewhere now that you're helping me."

* * * * *

Friday, August 7, 1981

At their second meeting the attorney confirmed that there were no provisions for a forced medical leave of absence.

"These medical staff bylaws provide only for a voluntary leave of absence, granted at a physician's request," Martin said. "In my opinion, the action taken against you resembles a summary suspension. The medical staff bylaws provide for a physician's clinical privileges to be summarily suspended by the hospital administrator whenever the physician, and I quote, 'has failed to carry out his professional responsibilities as set forth in these bylaws, rules, and regulations and the corporate bylaws of Hope Memorial Hospital, as well as any applicable departmental rules and regulations, so as to create a significant adverse effect on patient care,' end of quote. Where a practitioner's clinical privileges have been summarily suspended, the bylaws state that the practitioner is entitled to a hearing. I guess we'd better ask for a hearing right away."

Dr. Morgan was stunned. He had not realized the seriousness of the action against him and the complexities involved. He asked Martin, "Are you telling me that the action was improper, that they have to reinstate my privileges?"

"Not exactly," Martin replied. "What I'm saying is this: neither Dr. Thomas, Dr. Buchanan, nor White had any authority to impose a forced medical leave of absence on you according to the bylaws. Moreover, the action taken constitutes a summary suspension of your clinical privileges and you are therefore entitled to a hearing before an ad hoc committee of the medical staff for review of their action. However, you must request the hearing within 10 days after notification that your staff privileges have been suspended. If you don't make the request, you'll be deemed to have waived your right to a hearing. I believe it's been at least a week since you received that letter from the hospital. To get the hearing, you must request it very soon."

Dr. Morgan left the lawyer's office more confused and upset than when he had entered. He knew that in a hearing before an ad hoc committee, Dr. Thomas was likely to disclose the charges of professional misconduct raised against him. However, he felt that the only way to win reinstatement of his staff privileges at Hope Memorial would be to challenge his chief and White.

* * * * *

Saturday, August 8, 1981

Dr. Morgan sent a letter by messenger to the hospital, addressed to White, requesting a hearing in reference to the forced medical leave of absence that had been imposed upon him.

* * * * *

Monday, August 10, 1981

When the administrator saw the letter, he was not surprised by the request for a hearing. He suspected that Dr. Morgan had consulted an attorney and had been advised to seek such a review. He then called Drs. Thomas and Buchanan to his office to discuss the request.

"In my opinion, Dr. Morgan is entitled to a hearing under the medical staff bylaws," White said. "We need to get a committee together to decide whether the forced medical leave of absence is appropriate under the circumstances, if it is permissible under the bylaws, and whether Dr. Thomas was justified in rejecting Dr. Sanders's report and requiring instead an evaluation by Dr. Cooper."

White and Dr. Buchanan reviewed the procedure in the medical staff bylaws for the appointment of an ad hoc hearing committee. Dr. Buchanan, as president of the medical staff, was to appoint not fewer than five of its members to this committee. He gave White the names of five attending physicians from among several hospital departments, including medicine. His choice as chairman was Dr. Phillip Warner, an internist who also was the parliamentarian of the local county medical society. The physicians selected all were highly respected members of the medical staff whom Dr. Buchanan believed would fairly and impartially consider the Morgan situation.

White suggested that Dr. Buchanan, rather than he, contact them about their appointments. Dr. Buchanan reached all five by telephone and arranged to meet with them late that afternoon. When they had assembled in the hospital's board room, he told them, "I have selected you five to serve on an ad hoc hearing committee to investigate a forced medical leave of absence that has been instituted against a physician on the staff of the Department of Medicine. Service on this ad hoc committee is completely voluntary. The physician in question is Dr. John Morgan." He paused, then said, "Each of you should feel free to disqualify yourself from serving on the committee if a conflict of interest is presented."

Dr. Stephanie Fleming asked, "Can whatever problem exists be handled on an informal basis without establishing a special committee and conducting a formal hearing?"

"The medical staff bylaws guarantee the doctor a hearing once the doctor makes a request," Dr. Buchanan explained. "Dr. Morgan has submitted a written request for a hearing to Mr. White and, therefore, the hospital has no alternative but to grant it."

Dr. B.J. Adler commented, "There must be more than meets the eye here . . . .I saw him on the street just last night and he didn't look or act sick to me."

"I really don't want to get into the facts of the case at this time, but Dr. Morgan has recently been hospitalized and we felt we had no choice at this time but to impose this medical leave of absence," Dr. Buchanan answered.

"Would John Morgan really be likely to harm a patient if immediate steps had not been taken?" asked Dr. Louis Capolla.

Dr. Buchanan said quietly, "That possibility exists or else I wouldn't have gone along with the action. I am tempted to go into more detail with you, but I think we should curtail further discussion until all of you have agreed to serve on the committee."

After each agreed to serve and the five were attempting to clear dates, they continued to question Dr. Buchanan. He again avoided going into the facts of the case, saying, "I think we'd better wait until the hearing for more details. Mr. White will notify you of the date and location when we'll meet and, until then, I'm sure I don't need to caution you to maintain strict confidentiality. Mr. White is particularly concerned that we keep this matter private, both for Dr. Morgan's sake and for the sake of our entire staff's and the hospital's reputations."

* * * * *

Tuesday, August 11, 1981

White was able to schedule the hearing with less difficulty than he had expected, given the time of year. The administrator sent a letter by certified mail to Dr. Morgan, notifying him of the time, date, and place of the hearing. That letter contained Dr. Morgan's first official notification of the hospital's justification of its actions. White had attemped to phrase the statement of the charges very carefully:

> August 11, 1981
>
> Dear Dr. Morgan,
>
> As I have told you today by telephone, the hospital grants your request for a hearing related to your recent medical leave of absence. The hearing has been set for 8 A.M., August 24, 1981, in the board room at Hope Memorial.
>
> Recent events have led the Chief of Medicine, Dr. Ralph Thomas, to believe that you have become an impaired physician whose staff privileges have had to be curtailed in the best interests of the hospital, its patients, and yourself. Your recent illness and hospitalization caused the hospital administration to doubt whether your physical condition meets acceptable standards since you have refused to provide the requested medical report from your treating physician.
>
> In addition to providing facts about your hospitalization, you will be expected to respond to the following specific charges of professional incompetence: excessive drug orders for Demerol, failure to make regular patient rounds, failure to maintain proper patient charts, and failure to attend scheduled departmental and medical staff meetings and conferences.

> I quote from the medical staff bylaws that this hearing, "is for the purpose of intraprofessional resolution of the issues. Accordingly, neither the medical staff nor the practitioner shall be represented at the hearing by an attorney-at-law. Each party shall be entitled to be accompanied by a member of the medical staff in good standing."
> /s/*George White,* Administrator
> Hope Memorial Hospital

Now that the meeting was scheduled, White decided to telephone Paul Desberg, chairman of the Board of Trustees, to alert him to the Morgan situation, particularly that a hearing was to be held. After the administrator finished his recital of the events so far, Desberg commented, "This sounds like it could be a real sticky situation. I think you've done the right things so far, but why don't you touch base with Gordon Scott, the lawyer who handles most of the hospital's legal work? Gordon will be able to tell us how to handle this problem and where we should go from here."

When White called Scott, he was reluctant to go into much detail on the telephone, saying only that the medical staff was preparing to conduct a hearing on a physician, adding: "Since the hearing is scheduled to take place in a little less than two weeks, I want to meet with you as soon as possible in order to make certain that the hospital is following proper procedures."

White read Scott the letter he had sent to Dr. Morgan. Scott then recommended that they meet as soon as possible, before further correspondence was generated. "One wrong word can send you into a major lawsuit," he warned. They arranged a meeting at the hospital for the following morning.

* * * * *

Wednesday, August 12, 1981

White had compiled a "Dr. Morgan file" for his meeting with Scott. The file was very thin, reflecting the highly circumstantial nature of the hospital's evidence. It contained a few incident reports by nurses about the doctor's temper explosions and three letters from patients complaining about his inattentiveness to their repeated requests for medical reports or completion of insurance forms.

When Scott arrived, he was told about Dr. Morgan's collapse in the parking lot and the subsequent hospitalization. "This incident led me to discuss Dr. Morgan's situation in depth with his department chief, Dr. Ralph Thomas," White said.

"Oh, yes, he takes care of my sister," Scott commented.

"Um, well, Dr. Thomas described Dr. Morgan's erratic behavior. Then he told me about a disturbing report from the hospital pharmacist and quite a few specific incidents came up, although none of them are documented in the file. The big thing that happened—about two weeks ago—that triggered everything was the hospitalization. I learned that Dr. Thomas had confronted Dr. Morgan a while back. He also had made an informal agreement to keep quiet about Dr. Morgan's performance, and Dr. Morgan was supposed to shape up.

"One of our nurses, Linda Holmes, had access to Dr. Morgan's chart when he was over at East Side General. She took care of him in the ICU there and she couldn't understand why he wasn't responding to treatment for insulin shock until she saw his physician's note suggesting a drug or alcohol withdrawal reaction. She paid me a visit and gave me the story. She expected action, I should add.

"I put that together with what Dr. Thomas told me about the pharmacist's reports about his prescribing excess Demerol and the rest of it and decided to cancel his staff privileges, whatever way I could. We are holding the hearing on the 24th because that is within the three weeks from Dr. Morgan's request mentioned in the bylaws.

"One thing that concerns me is that some of the evidence may not be available, you know—confidentiality of patient records business and the reluctance of people to go on the record about others. What do you think?"

"Well, George," said the lawyer, "I'm a little concerned about the informal actions, or the lack of action, of Dr. Thomas several months ago. Of course, now we have the benefit of hindsight, but even so it seems as though the situation may have been serious enough at that time to warrant further investigation and action."

Scott looked up, startled, as White abruptly rose and began to pace agitatedly between his desk and the windows. The attorney then continued:

"I guess that's water under the bridge now, though. In light of Dr. Morgan's sudden hospitalization and inability to attend to his medical practice, the forced medical leave seems to be an appropriate step even though neither set of bylaws provides for it. I think it is reasonable for the hospital to require Dr. Morgan to submit complete medical reports from his treating physician before he is able to resume his hospital privileges."

White had stopped pacing and stood with his fingertips pressed on the desk top. He said, "Well, there's little doubt in my mind that Dr. Morgan has a problem and that we had to do something about it. What I'd have liked was to have the hospital assist a physician like this who suffers from drug addiction or another problem, but we can't gamble with the quality of patient care at the same time. I still want to help John Morgan. He'd been one of the top men in his department, but first he'll have to acknowledge his problem. If he won't admit to being a danger to his patients, we have no choice but to intercede on their behalf."

"I agree," Scott said, "and in my opinion, giving the doctor complete due process with respect to his request for a hearing on the matter is entirely correct. Even though there is no established procedure for instituting a forced medical leave of absence, the steps you took against Dr. Morgan we can treat as a summary suspension, for which he is entitled to a hearing in the bylaws. We'll follow those procedures for this hearing.

"With respect to the letter you have just sent to Dr. Morgan, outlining the charges against him, I'd like to take some time to review it carefully. We may need to supplement it with additional information. I'll look it over and get back to you. Meanwhile, I want to review with you the specific procedures in the bylaws for conducting the hearing. We better be certain that all procedures are followed. If we don't and the good doctor goes to court, the judge might ignore the fact that there was justification for yanking his ticket and put him back on the staff until he gets his proper hearing."

The attorney pulled some papers out of his briefcase and pulled his chair around so both men could look at the set of bylaws.

"Okay, a majority of the members of the hearing committee must be present when the hearing takes place and only those present may vote," Scott explained. "Dr. Morgan must be present at the hearing unless he waives his appearance or fails without good cause to appear. Dr. Morgan may be accompanied at the hearing by a member of the medical staff in good standing.

"You realize that if he has spoken to an attorney about this matter, there's a good chance the lawyer will want to attend this hearing with him. I know your bylaws don't provide for this but we may want to reconsider our position on this issue. There has been a New Jersey case where the court seemed to say that the hospital had denied the doctor due process by refusing to allow his attorney to be present during some hearing or review process. I'd better read that case and see how it might apply to our situation. Of course, we're not in New Jersey."

"Well, was I wrong to have already told Dr. Morgan that he couldn't be accompanied by an attorney?" asked White, with concern.

"No, not necessarily." Scott answered. "That's what the bylaws say, and we should stick with the procedures there unless they blatantly violate Dr. Morgan's rights. He may not even want an attorney present. Let's play that by ear.

"We also have to arrange to have an accurate record made of the hearing. You can either have a secretary take notes on the proceedings, or I can arrange to have a court reporter take down every word. I recommend the latter. We may need a complete record. It doesn't cost very much, and a verbatim record can be very useful if this ever gets to court.

"Dr. Warner is an excellent choice for chairman of the hearing committee. He knows parliamentary procedure almost as well as he knows medicine, maybe better. He'll preside, of course, determine the order of events, and keep everybody in line. I'll meet with him and advise him about how to handle procedural matters. One thing we have to keep in mind is that the scope of this hearing is strictly limited to the issues raised in the notice sent to Dr. Morgan. Dr. Warner should not allow any evidence in on an issue that Dr. Morgan has not been informed of in advance. Otherwise, he'll be able to claim he didn't have sufficient opportunity to prepare his defense."

"There's one thing I don't quite understand," the administrator said. "Do we have to prove our case against Dr. Morgan or does he have to prove his case against us? Who's on the defensive in this hearing?"

"Don't get this confused with a court of law," Scott replied. "This is more in line with an administrative agency proceeding. Dr. Morgan will have the burden of supporting his challenge by showing that the charges or grounds lack any factual basis or that the hospital's action is arbitrary, unreasonable, or capricious. We put that kind of language in the bylaws the last time we reviewed them, fortunately."

"Well," White said, "at least he'll be forced to deal with the drug issue then, since I specified the excessive Demerol orders in the letter I sent him."

"Right. As long as the issue was laid out in your letter, information can be presented as testimony regarding it," the lawyer answered. "Now, after the testimony is completed and the committee drafts its recommendation, I'd better take a look at it. Even though we may not allow lawyers to participate in the hearing, lawyers can assist the parties in their preparation."

White agreed, then decided to bring up the part of the Morgan problem he had been sitting on for two weeks. He asked Scott about the hospital's duty to report Dr. Morgan to the State Board of Medical Examiners as an impaired physician and how to handle Nurse Holmes's request for advice about her duty to report her suspicions. Scott seemed caught off guard.

"I am not too familiar with that," he said cautiously. "If we have such reporting laws, I'll look them over. In any event, I'll get back to you soon. Has anyone else talked to you about reporting to the state?"

White said, "No."

After Scott left, White sighed heavily. This would be his first experience with a medical staff hearing at Hope Memorial. He wondered if he should feel unlucky because of the Morgan problem or fortunate he hadn't had a serious physician issue before.

"Wouldn't it be better if Dr. Morgan would acknowledge his problem and get the necessary help?" he thought. He feared how the Morgan business would look in the newspaper, and how he'd look.

"How do I answer, if anyone asks the question, how long was Dr. Morgan on drugs before you did anything?" he thought. White realized he had a headache.

* * * * *

Wednesday, August 12, 1981

When Dr. Morgan received notice of the hearing, he became furious. He considered the specific items trivial. He also was disturbed that the hearing was scheduled for almost two weeks from his receipt of the notice. He telephoned White and demanded that they not wait the two weeks.

"Without hospital privileges, my practice is falling apart, you know that," he complained. "I'm perfectly sound both mentally and physically and I refuse to allow the hospital to take its own sweet time to ruin my career."

White listened politely. He told Dr. Morgan he would check with the members of the ad hoc committee and the others concerned, adding, "I'll be glad to move up the date of hearing if it can be conveniently arranged, John."

Dr. Morgan arranged to meet again with his lawyer. He showed Martin the notice of the hearing, then said, "I called George White and requested that he move up the date of the hearing. Did I do right?" Without pausing for an answer he went on, "They won't allow you to represent me at the hearing. I think it's unfair. The future of my medical career is on the line."

Martin nodded agreement and thought to himself, "It would be to Morgan's benefit to have an attorney at that hearing. He's acting really edgy and high-strung. He'll blow any chance he has." He also thought that the charges were too vague to prepare a proper response. After much discussion of the options, they agreed that Martin would prepare a letter to send to White.

* * * * *

Thursday, August 13, 1981

Martin sent the following letter:

> August 13, 1981
> Dear Mr. White,
> Please be informed that I have been retained to represent Dr. John Morgan in regard to the hearing to be held on the recommendation made by Dr. Ralph Thomas, Dr. James Buchanan, and you that Dr. Morgan's medical staff privileges be suspended. Please send me duplicate copies of any notices or communications that are directed to Dr. Morgan in connection with any of these proceedings.
> In the event that any of the records kept in the due course of business by the hospital, patient charts, or operating room notes are to be used in connection with the hearing, I request that true copies of same be sent to me prior to the hearing.

I do also request on behalf of Dr. Morgan a full and complete statement of the grounds for and the reasons why a decision was made to suspend his medical staff privileges, along with copies of any written communications that may have contained charges, complaints, or comments about Dr. Morgan's action or inactions that form the basis for said decision.

Dr. Morgan has provided me with a copy of your letter with the charges against him. I am shocked by their vague and obscure nature. In order for Dr. Morgan to prepare his defense for these charges, it will be absolutely necessary for him to be specifically informed as to the date or dates on which any incident or incidents are alleged to have occurred, and the particulars thereof.

Please transmit this information to me by return mail, and likewise transmit the information to Dr. Morgan so that we will have sufficient time to prepare an adequate response.

I also request on behalf of Dr. Morgan that the hospital reconsider its position on the presence of counsel at the hearing. Dr. Morgan is being denied due process of law under the bylaws of Hope Memorial Hospital and the United States Constitution in that he is not being afforded legal representation to assist him with his oral presentation and/or to answer any questions that may be presented.

I would also request to be informed of the names of the doctors appointed to the ad hoc committee that will hear this matter.

I will be happy to discuss this matter with you or any other hospital representative prior to the hearing date.

Very truly yours,

/s/*Peter Martin*

* * * * *

Friday, August 14, 1981

When White received the letter, he called Scott immediately and read it to him over the telephone. "Well, we knew this might happen," the attorney commented. "I'm a little concerned about the notice and I think I'll draft a supplemental notice for you to send to Dr. Morgan. Why don't you have his chief, Dr. Thomas, call me with specifics? I haven't had a chance to review that attorney case yet, but offhand I would recommend that you let him have his lawyer present. Nothing can be lost by having him there, and we will be taking a risk if you keep him out. Let's not give them any fuel for a fire."

White groaned. "The problem is this. I've discussed this matter with several members of the Medical Staff Executive Committee and the ad hoc hearing committee. With all due respect to you, you know these physicians have a thing about lawyers. They're afraid they'll be there all night if lawyers participate in the hearing. Besides, they feel strongly about adhering to the bylaws, since they wrote them. They think it's their document.''

''Well, there's no black-letter law about it in this state,'' Scott acknowledged carefully. ''But don't say I didn't warn you. If the problem with Dr. Morgan isn't resolved in a mutually satisfactory way and he takes the hospital to court, barring his attorney could come back to haunt you.''

After White spent several hours on the telephone to reschedule the hearing, he prepared and had delivered to Martin the following letter:

> August 14, 1981
> Dear Mr. Martin,
> Pursuant to the request of Dr. Morgan, we have changed the date of the hearing to August 18th at 7 P.M. in the board room of the Hope Memorial Hospital.
> The points contained in your letter have been considered. We are in the process of preparing a supplemental notice that will be delivered by messenger to you and Dr. Morgan this afternoon.
> Participation of attorneys at the hearing is not required by the bylaws and neither you nor the hospital's attorney will be permitted to attend the hearing. You may, however, assist Dr. Morgan in his preparation and wait outside the room during the hearing if you so desire. For further information concerning the hearing I suggest you consult the medical staff bylaws, a copy of which is enclosed.
> Very truly yours,
> /s/*George White*
> Administrator
> cc: Dr. John Morgan

* * * * *

Monday, August 17, 1981

The day before the scheduled date of the hearing, Dr. Buchanan distributed a packet of materials to the five members of the hearing committee and to Dr. Thomas and Dr. Morgan. The packet included the following items: Written statements by Dr. Thomas and David Gormon, director of pharmacy, summarizing their knowledge and observations concerning Dr. Morgan; copies of incident reports filed by various nurses; copies of letters of complaint received by the hospital from patients of Dr. Morgan; an unsigned statement on the letterhead of East Side General Hospital acknowledging that Dr. Morgan was an inpatient there from July 25 to July 30; a copy of the Carey Ambulance

Service Call Report, which noted that Dr. Morgan was transferred in a comatose state, with numerous track marks on his arms, from King's Liquor Store parking lot to East Side General Hospital; and a copy of a letter addressed "To Whom It May Concern" from Dr. Mark Sanders attesting to Dr. Morgan's good state of health.

Copies of the relevant sections of the medical staff bylaws titled "Corrective Action" and "Hearing and Appellate Review Procedures" also were distributed, along with copies of all correspondence and notices between the hospital and Dr. Morgan and his attorney.

* * * * *

Tuesday, August 18, 1981

The hearing committee was convened as scheduled at 7 P.M. Present were all the members of the committee, Dr. Morgan, Dr. Thomas, Gormon, White, and a court reporter obtained by the hospital.

Dr. Warner, chairman of the hearing committee, presided. He introduced the committee members and read into the record the letter imposing the medical leave and the correspondence containing the charges that were to be considered. Dr. Warner also reviewed the procedures that would be followed and concluded by stating:

"At the conclusion of the presentation of the oral and written evidence by both sides, and after each side has had the opportunity to present its case, those parties shall leave the room and the hearing committee shall deliberate in closed session. This committee shall submit its findings and recommendations to the Medical Staff Executive Committee, which will review our recommendations and will make its recommendation to the Board of Trustees. The Board of Trustees has the final decision in this matter."

The testimony opened with a long statement by Dr. Thomas, who described the instances of Dr. Morgan's conduct that had been brought to his attention for more than a year. Specifically, the chief of medicine mentioned Dr. Morgan's failure to make regular patient rounds, his confused and overlong patient chart entries, failure to send patient records to other physicians upon request, failure to complete patient insurance forms, failure to keep scheduled appointments with patients, and his inability to get along with the staff nurses and other hospital personnel.

In some instances Dr. Thomas cited specific examples of these shortcomings but frequently he spoke in generalities. He explained that he was laying the groundwork for his ultimate conclusion that Dr. Morgan was an impaired physician. He then briefly described his meeting with Gormon, the hospital's pharmacist. He indicated that Gormon would provide a more detailed account of the Pharmacy Department's review of Dr. Morgan's prescribing pattern.

Dr. Thomas then described his meeting with Dr. Morgan and the informal agreement they had reached in which he agreed not to seek formal disciplinary action, provided that Dr. Morgan improved his professional conduct. The medical chief said this was one of the most difficult problems he had ever faced. He was sympathetic to the fact that Dr. Morgan at that time was disturbed over his son's death and it was for that reason alone that he was willing to give him a second chance.

Dr. Thomas detailed the incident in the liquor store parking lot and Dr. Morgan's subsequent hospitalization at East Side General. He felt that the situation now amounted to an emergency, so he wholeheartedly supported imposing a forced medical leave of absence on Dr. Morgan and insisting that Dr. Seymour Cooper, Dr. Morgan's regular treating physician, submit a complete report on his patient's present physical health before even considering allowing resumption of his privileges at Hope Memorial. Dr. Thomas steadfastly maintained that Dr. Sanders's letter stating that Dr. Morgan was in good physical health was inadequate under the circumstances. He said:

"Dr. Sanders is a general practitioner in a community 25 miles away who examined Dr. Morgan on only this one occasion. On the other hand, Dr. Cooper has treated Dr. Morgan for the past several years. He would be familiar with Dr. Morgan's diabetic condition and his condition during his hospitalization at East Side General, the event which triggered our decision to require a forced medical leave of absence. I feel we are making a reasonable request although Dr. Morgan has reacted with rage and scorn to our reasonable and appropriate condition for reinstatement."

As Dr. Thomas spoke, Dr. Morgan sat looking balefully at him and the other men who had signed the letter to him. He nearly leaped to his feet several times but restrained himself. Dr. Thomas concluded, "In summary, my mounting suspicions concerning Dr. Morgan, substantiated by the discovery of multiple track marks on his arms, led me to believe that the hospital would be acting reasonably and prudently in forcing Dr. Morgan to accept a medical leave of absence."

Dr. Morgan then was given the opportunity to question Dr. Thomas. As he rose to his full height of 5 feet 6 inches and paced across the room, he asked Dr. Thomas sarcastically whether he had any evidence that was neither rumor nor hearsay. Dr. Thomas replied:

"The general consensus of all concerned was that the quality of your patient care was deteriorating and all signs pointed to only one cause. The floor nurses who voiced complaints regarding your professional conduct are reluctant to serve as witnesses out of fear of retaliatory action from you or other physicians. Also, as I understand the bylaws, the nurses' testimony is not necessary since formal rules of evidence need not be followed."

Dr. Morgan argued to the committee that some of those complaints were more than a year old. He noted that he had been recommended for reappointment, after endorsement by Dr. Thomas, just three months before. "Surely," he said, "my reappointment has wiped the slate clean as far as those minor complaints were concerned. No doctor in this hospital is perfect. These prima donna nurses should have more important things to do, like taking care of patients, instead of checking what time I make rounds. You can't force a man off the staff for this nonsense."

Dr. Morgan paused, then practically shouted, "My practice is being destroyed by invisible enemies. They're jealous of my success and they're ashamed to come forward in public to repeat their lies and insinuations."

Dr. Warner, the chairman, soothed him by saying, "The committee will bear in mind the sources of the allegations when we deliberate on the issues before us."

Gormon's testimony followed. The pharmacist told the panel:

"My suspicions regarding Dr. Morgan were initially aroused when a routine drug audit revealed that he was prescribing Demerol for nearly all of his patients, regardless of the admitting diagnosis. Moreover, Dr. Morgan frequently reordered Demerol even when the patient was able to swallow and was being administered other medications orally.

"After I studied the audit, I decided to speak to some floor nurses about Dr. Morgan's patients in an effort to determine whether their conditions warranted the intravenous administration of Demerol and whether the patients exhibited the usual side effects of this drug, such as nausea and hypotension. I was told that the majority of Dr. Morgan's patients who were receiving Demerol were taking other medications orally, although they had IVs running, and that they were not exhibiting the customary side effects of Demerol.

"After talking with the floor nurses and reviewing Dr. Morgan's patients' charts, I had decided to track his drug orders for several weeks before approaching Dr. Thomas about what I suspected. I found that Dr. Morgan continued to prescribe Demerol for many patients even though the need for administering the drug intravenously appeared questionable. I suspected that, in actuality, many of these patients were not receiving this medication. I tried to speak to Dr. Morgan about his unusual drug prescribing habits on a few occasions, but when I did he was furious; he absolutely refused to discuss the matter, and he threatened to have me fired. At that point, I felt that I had no alternative but to inform Dr. Thomas of my suspicions."

He added, "Diabetics like Dr. Morgan are more likely to abuse drugs via self-injection than any other form of self-administration."

The members of the committee were noticeably impressed by Gormon's testimony, which appeared to lend substantive credence to Dr. Thomas's statements.

Dr. Morgan was barely able to control his anger. When Gormon had finished, Dr. Morgan asked sarcastically, "When have pharmacists been licensed to practice medicine and to decide whether a specific drug was medically necessary in a specific situation?" He then asked the committee, "How can you pay any attention to him? Why aren't doctors testifying about my orders? Why are no patients' charts referred to specifically?"

Dr. Morgan paused, then faced the committee and said, "I'm inclined to walk out of this hearing right now. This is unbelievable!"

Dr. Warner tried to calm Dr. Morgan. "If you would like a recess, Dr. Morgan, we'll all agree to take a break."

"No, never mind," Dr. Morgan muttered, "let's get this mud-slinging over with. Bring on some more garbage!"

The hearing proceeded. White, Hope Memorial's administrator, testified how he learned from Dr. Post of Dr. Morgan's collapse in the liquor store parking lot and his subsequent hospitalization at East Side General. He explained that he had immediately made arrangements, with the assistance of Dr. Thomas, for the care of Dr. Morgan's patients who were then in the hospital. White went on:

"At that time Dr. Thomas informed me of the serious situation that had developed concerning Dr. Morgan's professional conduct at Hope Memorial. I talked with Bill Connors, the administrator of East Side General, and Dr. Cooper, Dr. Morgan's treating physician, on the Monday after Dr. Morgan's admission to East Side General, and I was quite frustrated by both of those conversations. I believe that both Connors and Dr. Cooper knew a great deal more than they were saying.

"You know, I appreciate a patient's right to confidentiality, but I felt that more important issues were at stake in this matter. At any rate, I was unable to obtain any specific information from Connors and Dr. Cooper. Connors merely agreed to confirm in writing the dates on which Dr. Morgan was admitted to and discharged from East Side General."

White paused. He then announced that he had irrefutable evidence that Dr. Morgan's own physician had acknowledged the probable drug problem and that this evidence had come to light without a breach of confidentiality by Dr. Cooper. He told the committee of his visit from a reliable nurse who was employed at Hope Memorial and who occasionally moonlighted at East Side General.

"She was working the evening shift in the Intensive Care Unit of East Side General the day that Dr. Morgan was admitted there," he said. "Although the admitting diagnosis on Dr. Morgan had been insulin shock, this nurse told me that he failed to respond to standard treatment for the diagnosed condition. She also said that an entry on Dr. Morgan's medical chart by Dr. Cooper indicated that Dr. Cooper suspected that his patient was suffering from a drug withdrawal reaction."

White paused again, then explained, "The purpose of this nurse's visit to me was to inquire about her legal duty to report Dr. Morgan to the state as an impaired physician."

The committee was very intent as White continued:

"In light of all this and other incriminating information I had received, together with the fact that Dr. Morgan was hospitalized and unavailable to take care of patients, I felt that the hospital had no choice but to impose a forced medical leave of absence on him. When I told Dr. Thomas and Dr. Buchanan, we agreed that it would be irresponsible to delay action until the Medical Staff Executive Committee's next meeting, which was scheduled for several weeks later. We felt that the committee could cancel or modify the leave of absence if it determined that our action was inappropriate or uncalled for."

White concluded his testimony by asserting, "I fully supported Dr. Thomas's decision not to accept Dr. Sanders's report in lieu of a report from Dr. Cooper."

Dr. Morgan was astounded. The packet of material he had received from Dr. Buchanan before the hearing contained very few references to his stay at East Side General and no mention at all of a nurse in the East Side ICU reporting having seen Dr. Cooper's entries on his chart. He had gone over the packet thoroughly with his attorney, who had tried to show him some of the weaknesses and holes in the hospital's preparation.

He was totally unprepared for this testimony concerning the note on his chart. He had assumed that any information concerning his stay at East Side General was confidential. He did not have any idea who his nurse had been while he was unconscious but he silently swore at her loose tongue. Dr. Morgan did not ask White a single question. Instead, he made a short speech to the committee, saying "All you've heard is gossip, innuendo, and hearsay. There's not one shred of cold, hard proof that has been put before you in this hearing. Just talk."

It was then Dr. Morgan's turn to present his case. He adamantly denied that he was addicted to any drug, and specifically Demerol. He declared:

"It is necessary for me to take insulin daily in order to control my diabetes, but this is the only medication I use regularly. It is sometimes necessary for me to inject the insulin into my arms. This explains the needle tracks that have been reported. My absences from departmental meetings and staff conferences were attributable to my personal problems. Can't you consider the tremendous stress and anxiety to which I have been subjected? My son committed suicide last year and my ex-wife suffered a nervous breakdown over it."

His face showed the strain as he went on, saying, "Despite the extreme pressure I have been under throughout this period, I have never been lax or negligent in the care of my patients. In fact, I maintain that my conduct at the hospital has steadily improved.''

He acknowledged his hospitalization at East Side General but explained that the initial failure of the treatment was attributable to the unusually low level of sugar in his blood, since he apparently had administered too much insulin that day.

''I fail to understand,'' he said, ''why Dr. Thomas should be able to insist upon a letter from a physician who no longer treats me. I had a professional disagreement with Dr. Cooper and I sought out a new personal physician. Since I am now under Dr. Sanders's care, a statement from him concerning my present physical health is completely appropriate. After all, Dr. Thomas is supposedly concerned with my current physical health and my present ability to resume work at the hospital. Therefore, this insistence upon a report from Dr. Cooper is simply a means to accomplish the goal of destroying my career.

''The allegations of professional misconduct are groundless. I wish I knew who all of these individuals are who are out to ruin my career at Hope Memorial by alleging that I am addicted to drugs. I question the validity of the evidence that has been presented to the ad hoc committee. I demand to know how the committee can rely upon the medical expertise of the hospital pharmacist, presented without any patient charts in support of his claims, when obviously the hospital can find no physicians who are willing to support Gormon's lay judgment and far-fetched conclusions.

''Every man has the constitutional right to be confronted by his accusers and yet my career is being maliciously destroyed by lies, innuendo, and hearsay. I request the committee to be impartial in its deliberations and I want to point out that if anyone is out to get you, you could find yourself in a similar situation to mine.''

The members of the committee were very attentive to Dr. Morgan's last comment and his point hit a responsive chord.

With Dr. Morgan's statement completed, the members of the ad hoc committee questioned the witnesses. Dr. Howard Cook asked whether the committee would see a copy of the latest ''Attestation of Health'' from the Medical Staff Executive Committee's file on Dr. Morgan. Every physician at Hope was required to fill out this questionnaire as part of the hospital's annual reappointment process. Dr. Buchanan, president of the medical staff, had a copy that he passed around the committee. It revealed that Dr. Morgan had made no reference to his use of any drug, including insulin. Dr. Buchanan acknowledged, however, that the questionnaire asked only whether the applicant was then under the care of another physician for any medical problem.

Dr. Morgan asked to see the copy of the ''Attestation of Health'' report he had signed. He read to the committee the following language from the bottom of the document: ''I have reviewed the physical and mental health status of Dr.

Morgan. Based on my review I recommend that Dr. Morgan be reappointed for the next medical staff year.'' He added, ''This statement was signed by Dr. Thomas.''

Dr. Cook asked,''Well, Dr. Thomas,why did you sign this if you had doubts about Dr. Morgan's health and suspected him of abusing Demerol? Couldn't you have forced him to submit to a physical before you reappointed him?''

Dr. Thomas answered, ''You know, I forgot all about this statement. I think it was a JCAH requirement that I sign one for each member of my department. Besides, Dr. Morgan and I had struck an informal bargain and I suppose I felt obligated to give him a chance. In retrospect, if I had taken advantage of this opportunity to substantiate my suspicions, we might not have so much trouble and bitterness as we have now.''

Committee members asked whether Dr. Thomas would automatically reinstate Dr. Morgan if he provided a letter from Dr. Cooper. The chief of medicine replied that if the letter addressed the drug use issue in a satisfactory manner, then he would consider reinstatement. He also said that if Dr. Morgan would agree to acknowledge his problem and seek appropriate treatment, a compromise could be worked out in which the physician's confidentiality would be protected. He added, ''Listen, my ultimate objective has been to help, not ruin, Dr. Morgan, but I can't do this without Dr. Morgan's admitting he knows of his problem.''

When all of the committee's questions had been answered, Dr. Warner adjourned the hearing, stating that the panel would meet privately and issue its conclusions within the next few days.

''What?'' Dr. Morgan cried. ''You're going to continue this hearing without me? You can't do that. I'm entitled to stay in this room until you reach a decision. Besides, you'd better reach a decision right now. I've got patients who I want to admit to my service. I'm tired of referring around. If you won't see fit to give me back my hospital privileges, my lawyer and I will get you in court.''

''Calm down, John,'' Dr. Warner said. ''We want to resolve this issue as quickly as you do. But it's after 10 o'clock now, and we've all had long days. As for myself, I'd like to digest the testimony I've heard here today before arriving at a decision. I don't want to be rushed into a decision I might regret later. I think we all feel that suspending any fellow physician's privileges is a serious matter and is a responsibility we aren't taking lightly.

''If the committee agrees, I'm willing to stay for an additional hour to see if we can arrive at a decision. However, neither you nor anyone else will be permitted to be present while we deliberate. The bylaws don't provide for that.

Noting that several members of the committee nodded approvingly, Dr. Warner said, ''I think that is a good idea and I suggest we consider it as one of our alternatives.''

and, besides, we should have the opportunity to discuss this matter openly and freely without having any outsiders present. Does the committee have any objections?''

None were expressed.

''All right,'' Dr. Warner said, ''let's start discussing this and see how far we get. Will everyone except the members of the committee please leave the room?''

Dr. Morgan was muttering as he stormed out, heading for the pay telephone to call his attorney.

* * * * *

The committee members then began their deliberations. All of the members sensed that Dr. Morgan was trying to conceal something and that he might very well be suffering from a drug problem, although the seriousness of the situation was not entirely clear. Most of the group acknowledged that much of the evidence was circumstantial in nature but they felt that it combined to create a strong presumption that Dr. Morgan's denials had failed to overcome.

Dr. Warner reminded the committee that, under the bylaws, the burden was on Dr. Morgan to show that the hospital's charges lacked any factual basis and that the forced medical leave of absence was arbitrary, unreasonable, and capricious. The members were especially concerned that Dr. Morgan had not directly denied Gormon's statements about the volume of his Demerol orders. Equally damaging was White's testimony about the entry in the East Side General chart that suggested Dr. Morgan's probable drug addiction.

The committee agreed that Dr. Morgan should provide Dr. Thomas with a report from Dr. Cooper. The panel felt this request was reasonable because it was Dr. Morgan's collapse and subsequent hospitalization at East Side General that prompted the temporary suspension of his privileges at Hope Memorial.

At this point, Dr. Fleming said, ''I have the apprehension that the rest of you have about Dr. Morgan's responses to the charges made against him and I feel that we must take some action to protect the hospital and its patients. But I wonder if there isn't some action we can take that would, in effect, remove his privileges without resorting to a suspension and the stigma attached to that.''

''Like what?'' Dr. Warner asked.

''Well,'' Dr. Fleming answered, ''could we recommend to Dr. Morgan that he apply for a voluntary leave of absence? Of course, we would probably want him to make some unofficial acknowledgement of his problem to the committee. That would permit him to save face. It would protect the hospital and its patients and, not incidentally, would save the hospital from the possibility that Dr. Morgan will bring a suit against it.''

* * * * *

Wednesday, August 19, 1981

The morning after the hearing, Dr. Warner drafted the committee's written report and recommendations and circulated it to the members for comment. Two days later a final report was sent to the president of the medical staff, Dr. Buchanan. Neither the draft nor the final version was shown to the hospital's attorney, Scott.

The report stated that the committee found that the hospital had not acted unreasonably in its actions. It recommended that a complete report on Dr. Morgan's hospitalization and physical health be submitted by Dr. Cooper as a condition for lifting the forced medical leave of absence.

It also recommended that as an alternative, Dr. Morgan be given the opportunity to acknowledge his drug abuse problem confidentially and unofficially and be granted a voluntary leave of absence to obtain appropriate treatment and counseling. After evidence of his rehabilitation was presented, his leave of absence would be terminated and he would be permitted to resume his medical staff privileges.

* * * * *

Wednesday, August 26, 1981

The committee's report was received by Dr. Buchanan in time for the regular meeting of the Medical Staff Executive Committee on August 26. Fortunately, enough members were in the city to make a quorum.

When Dr. Buchanan convened the meeting he said an urgent matter involving a summary suspension would be first on the agenda. He added that, although he had brought about the action, he would preside. He said a hearing already had been held. Most of the committee members evidently knew a good deal about the Morgan situation already judging by the knowing glances exchanged. One member asked whether they were obliged to accept the recommendations of the ad hoc committee because he wanted to know whether they could develop another solution.

Dr. Buchanan responded that the recommendations of the hearing committee were not binding on the Medical Staff Executive Committee.

"Then why did you bother to have a hearing in the first place?" the physician asked.

Dr. Buchanan, annoyed, said, "Let's not get sidetracked. Why don't we review and discuss the report before we decide anything?"

After some discussion, the group voted to accept the ad hoc committee report and recommendations and White was so informed. Under the medical staff bylaws, the administrator was responsible for giving Dr. Morgan prompt written notice of the decision.

* * * * *

Thursday, August 27, 1981

The next morning White drafted a letter to Dr. Morgan to inform him of the results of the Medical Staff Executive Committee meeting.

White called Scott, Hope Memorial's attorney, to review his draft letter. Scott reminded him to include notice of Dr. Morgan's right to appeal the decision to the hospital's Board of Trustees as well as a copy of the hearing committee's report. He said this report would be helpful to Dr. Morgan and his lawyer, Martin, in deciding whether to appeal the decision. White mailed copies of the letter and report to Dr. Morgan's home, his private office, and to Martin's office.

* * * * *

Friday, August 28, 1981

Dr. Morgan anxiously awaited word from the hospital. His practice was dwindling, so he had to inform his patients that he was going on sabbatical and would not be available to see them for a while. When the letter and report arrived, they shocked him into action. He telephoned Martin in panic.

"Oh, God, my medical practice is destroyed and my privileges at Hope Memorial will never be reinstated," he moaned. "Do you think we ought to take them to court?"

Martin tried to allay his client's fears by pointing out all the options that still were left to him. He added, "I think we ought to discuss this in person, Dr. Morgan. Can you make it to my office in an hour and a half?"

"Of course, of course, I'll be there. Good-bye."

When Dr. Morgan walked into the attorney's office his face was pale and his hands trembled. He had expected to be reinstated; he felt betrayed by old friends. He sat hunched in the huge, brown leather wing chair that Martin reserved for visitors, waiting for some hopeful words. Without his anger to buoy him, he seemed drained of energy and his small frame seemed to have shrunk even further. As Martin began to talk, he leaned forward to concentrate.

"Dr. Morgan, I do not think we ought to consider litigation yet. It's premature. The bylaws provide you with the opportunity to appeal the Medical Staff Executive Committee's adverse recommendation. I think you ought to request that appeal. It would, at least, keep pressure on the hospital and preserve all your options. You see, we have to play by the rules in the bylaws before you can begin litigation."

"I don't think you realize what all this means to me, Pete," Morgan said. "I've already told a number of my patients that I'm going on sabbatical, to save face, but by the time we appeal, my practice will be just about finished. And if that goes against me and I do sue, I'm afraid I'll never be able to practice in town here. There'll be no practice left to save! I'm no youngster; I can't start all over."

"Look, you still have options," Martin said. "In addition to the appeal, you still can go to Dr. Cooper. If he examines you and reports that you're capable of resuming practice at Hope Memorial, according to what Dr. Thomas has said, he will rescind this forced medical leave of absence. You could be back in business very shortly."

Martin watched his client carefully as he spoke. What he saw caused him to pause. The physician sat quite still, dwarfed by the big chair, and tears trickled slowly down his lined cheeks. Martin went on:

"Dr. Morgan, if you don't choose that option, you could still accept the hospital's conditions for a voluntary leave of absence. I'm a little wary of that route, since it means you must acknowledge that you have a drug problem. Although it's unlikely that you would be subject to any criminal action even if your so-called confidential, unofficial admission ever becomes public, I can't guarantee that you won't be the target of civil suits or an administrative hearing. What that could mean, ultimately, I'm afraid, is suspension or revocation of your license to practice medicine."

After a long silence, Dr. Morgan said very softly, "Would you please contact the Board of Trustees for me to request the appeal?"

He straightened his shoulders, looking more dignified, and said, "I'm afraid I may not have been a very good client, Pete. Until after the hearing, I really thought I'd get this thing to blow over." He reached into his jacket pocket for a handkerchief, wiped his cheeks, and blew his nose. "I will make an appointment to see Seymour Cooper next week and let you know what happens."

As the two men stood and shook hands, Martin noted that his client had stopped trembling and realized, with some relief, that the session had gone quite well—no fireworks. Facing the physician, he spoke sympathetically, "Dr. Morgan, I believe we have a good chance of resolving this promptly. I hope all goes well when you see Dr. Cooper, but if he doesn't help you to make a simple end to it, we do still have the appeal to the board, as you know."

As he spoke, he became aware of a change in Dr. Morgan's handclasp and glanced up to see renewed tension in the lines over his client's eyes. He realized that Dr. Morgan felt he was a beaten man. To Dr. Morgan, following the procedures in the hospital's bylaws had strung out the situation over time so that unless he went to court and won a sizeable judgment (a very unlikely possibility), his problem had created professional and financial disaster for him.

"Well, anyway," Martin said as he patted Dr. Morgan on the shoulder, "I'll be available if you need me. Phone me after you've seen Dr. Cooper."

* * * * *

Monday, August 31, 1981

When Dr. Morgan arrived for his appointment with Dr. Cooper he was subdued. He thought, "If Seymour doesn't come through, I'm just going to plead with Ralph Thomas. He'll have to help me now."

As Dr. Cooper entered the examination room, Dr. Morgan said, trying to be casual, "Well, Seymour, I'm here for another physical. I know you've seen me recently during that episode in the hospital, but this time it's a matter of getting me back on the staff at Hope Memorial. My chief has imposed a temporary medical leave on me because of that hospitalization and he wants a complete report from you before he'll reinstate me. I hope you'll give me a clean bill of health so I can get back to work."

Dr. Morgan did not mention the hearing or the Medical Staff Executive Committee's decision to continue the forced leave of absence. He didn't know how much, if anything, Dr. Cooper knew about the events at Hope but he feared the worst.

Before beginning to examine Dr. Morgan, Dr. Cooper said gravely:

"John, we've known each other for more than a few years now. Let's be honest with one another. Your collapse at the liquor store parking lot was totally unrelated to your diabetes. I've suspected for some time that you have a drug problem, although I never had the necessary lab tests or results to prove it. When I treated you at East Side General my suspicions were confirmed. First there were the needle marks. Then your symptoms on admission indicated insulin shock and I ordered standard therapy for that condition, but you failed to respond to the treatment. The symptoms continued and, in fact, they were alleviated only after the drug withdrawal was complete.

"John, you're a physician. You know as well as I do that a severe drug withdrawal reaction can strongly resemble insulin shock. I know you have been under a great deal of stress and tension during the past several months and I know that the divorce and suicide have not been easy for you.

"As a doctor and, I hope, a friend, I have to tell you that I sincerely believe you must recognize and admit that you do have a drug problem, and that you must seek rehabilitation. I know of similar cases where the physicians involved did seek therapy and they were able to kick their drug habits. I know you can, too, if you want to. The choice is yours. I don't need to examine you. You have to examine yourself. I can't say you can practice as if nothing happened. I'll work with you. I'll talk to the folks at Hope. Just let's not kid ourselves any more."

Dr. Morgan replied, "Seymour, I'm not going to plead with you. I did think that our long professional and personal relationship would have some effect on your decision about this, though."

"Well, John, in a way it has. If it weren't for our long history together I might have questioned you earlier and had this confirmed before you had to be brought in to that emergency room. I'm sorry for the part I've played in delaying this, more than you realize. As your physician and your friend, I'm refusing to allow you to continue on a path that can lose you your license and your dignity, to say nothing about your health."

"Forgive me if I yearn for a little less friendship," Dr. Morgan answered sarcastically. "I'd prefer the opportunity to get back to work immediately. I suppose I knew this would come sometime, though I've tried my damndest to avoid it. Tell me, Seymour, what chance do you think I'll have of regaining any kind of practice in three or six months?"

His face showed both anger and despair.

"John, I just don't know, but I'll tell you one thing. I think you'll be surprised by the kind of cooperation the other men will give you when they see what you're trying to do to improve your life. I think you can build it up again. After all, you've always had a fine reputation."

"God, I hope you're right," Dr. Morgan said. "I hope you're right."

"Well, John, I'll stand by you in any way I can that will help you get back on your feet."

"Thanks, Seymour. If you're sure I can't make some sort of deal now, I may have to call on you for some help later. I guess that's it."

Dr. Morgan rose, shook hands with Dr. Cooper, and left the office.

Forgetting about calling his lawyer, he phoned Dr. Thomas from a pay telephone on the corner. He told himself that he had to get this over with before he had time to think about it.

"Dr. Thomas, this is John Morgan. I'd like to come in to see you in about 20 minutes, if possible. You can? Good, I'll be right over."

* * * * *

Dr. Morgan attemped to strike a bargain with Dr. Thomas. He said he would ask Dr. Cooper to help him enroll in a drug treatment program and that he would promise not to appeal to the board or bring a lawsuit against Hope Memorial, if he was put on voluntary leave of absence status.

"What I also need from you is a promise, in writing this time, that you will keep the matter secret and confidential, and that you will automatically reinstate me once I complete the therapy," he said.

With great relief Dr. Thomas answered, "I promise to do all I can to help your rehabilitation efforts. I will have to check with George White first, particularly about anything being put in writing, I'm almost positive that we can work this out. Congratulations, John, this is a big step for you and I'm sure you're on the right road."

Dr. Thomas called White promptly to tell the administrator about the visit. They agreed to recommend in principle acceptance of Dr. Morgan's request at a special Medical Staff Executive Committee meeting that was to be held the following week. White said, "You know, I believe it's in everyone's best interest to specify that all the records of this whole matter be sealed. I want to confirm our planned course of action with Gordon Scott and the chairman of the board."

White then called Scott with great enthusiasm to bring the hospital's attorney up to date. He spoke at length without interruption, ending by asking, "Gordon, how will these recent developments affect our duty to report Dr. Morgan to the state as an impaired physician?"

"Hold on, that's a matter that was way down on the priority scale," Scott replied. "I've not intruded very much. Actually you and the others have involved me very little. But now I feel I must be more involved. Nothing is to be put in writing without my approval. I suppose I can work with Dr. Morgan's lawyer. What has gone on is what you people call 'resolving something on an intraprofessional basis.' Well, when it comes to putting a deal down on paper, it's a matter for another profession, the legal profession. Whether a report is made is an open question. I'll look into it and give you my advice on that soon. Overall, I think the deal is a decent one."

"You'd better!" White responded. "I think we need to know the answer about the report, though, because it affects the commitment to Dr. Morgan for confidentiality."

"Well," Scott said, "if the nurse who came to you will agree to keep confidential what she knows, and if Dr. Morgan isn't seeing any patients during this entire time, even if this technically is something to report, we probably won't do it. But I want to check it out."

"That Nurse Holmes is a hard nose," White said. "Are you suggesting that the deal, as you put it, depends on her going along?"

"Perhaps," Scott answered. "There's something for you to work on."

After the conversation ended, White called in his secretary and said, "Find out if Linda Holmes, a nurse, is in the house now. If she is, call her for me."

A few minutes later his secretary buzzed and said that Nurse Holmes was on the line. White pressed the button to connect with the nurse and said, "Linda, I want to speak with you about our conversation of a few weeks ago. Could you join me for dinner this evening at the University Club?"

Commentary

1.

Many times a medical staff problem seems to drag on beyond the point of an apparent resolution. Tying up loose ends, to put the matter entirely to rest, presents the hospital's executive and key members of the medical staff with additional responsibilities. In this case study, the question of whether a report to the State Board of Medical Examiners will be made is not finally answered. Furthermore, if the physician, Dr. Morgan, participates in a rehabilitation program, there is no guarantee that he will necessarily be successful and the hospital may find itself in the position of having to refuse to terminate the medical leave of absence. Unfortunately, solutions to medical staff problems cannot be neatly packaged and readily concluded in many instances, a circumstance that has to be accepted.

2.

The medical staff bylaws did not provide a procedure that exactly matched what the hospital administrator believed needed to be done in the case study. As carefully drawn as those bylaws may be, there always is the possibility that a set of events will occur that does not fall into a specific cubbyhole established in the hospital's or medical staff's documents.

Although this can be disconcerting, board members, administrators, and medical staff leaders must recognize that, because of the responsibilities imposed on hospitals by state laws and regulations, there is authority of an inherent nature to permit the institution to deal with problems for which it has responsibility, even if it is necessary to establish ad hoc procedures.

When this is done, there is a possibility that, if the matter reaches a court, the judge will be concerned about the failure to function exactly in accord with the hospital documents. Hospital counsel should be able to make clear in such a situation the need for the action taken. If the physician involved has been granted the hearing and appeal rights generally provided in the documents, and the institution has a supportable substantive case, it should be successful in court.

It is imperative in such situations that the advice of the hospital attorney be sought promptly. In the case study the hospital attorney was not brought into the situation until the basic framework for what would follow already had been established, and only after the suggestion to involve him was made by the president of the board. While it does not appear that this failure to consult the attorney created any impediment to the handling of the matter, it might have alleviated, if not eliminated, the anxiety that the hospital administrator had regarding the proper way to proceed.

With respect to the role of the attorney in the case study as a whole, it would appear that it was not major at any point. In situations of the nature described, there is the potential for the hospital attorney to contact the physician's lawyer before the initial formal proceeding. Given the sensitivity of the impaired physician problem, an attempt ordinarily should be made to negotiate an arrangement that will spare the hospital some difficulty and spare the physician the discomfort of the issues being aired through a formal process.

3.

Dr. Thomas, the chief of medicine, is shown in the case study to have procrastinated after he became aware of Dr. Morgan's difficulties by failing to take any decisive action. There is a tendency in the medical profession to temporize when a physician with problems, who previously had been a respected member of the medical staff and a competent practitioner, evidences serious difficulties. There is the hope—rarely an expectation, though—that the situation will be cleared up without decisive action.

Understandably, granting the physician an opportunity to reform is an attractive approach to a professional colleague. The problem is that it is a route taken too often without even notification of other key persons in the medical staff, or the hospital's executive. It might very well be argued that the department chairman should not make such decisions without the advice and concurrence of others. In the case study, if Dr. Morgan had not collapsed and been hospitalized, it is quite possible that his erratic and poor performance would have continued indefinitely without any action by the hospital.

The purpose of the department chairman's recommendation regarding reappointment is to provide a candid evaluation of the physician's past performance, and the prospect for the coming year, at the level required by the hospital. To ignore this responsibility not only is to do a disservice to the hospital but also is to lay the basis for a successful lawsuit against the institution and, perhaps, the department chairman individually, if a patient suffers harm caused by the services of the physician who has received a favorable recommendation from his chairman, notwithstanding reasons calling for a negative report, and is reappointed. There already have been sufficient court decisions dealing with failures in medical staff processes to acknowledge poor performance of staff physicians to make clear the liability potential in these situations.

4.

Statutes requiring reports of hospital disciplinary actions against physicians, impaired physicians, and malpractice awards or settled claims are on the increase. These so-called "tattletale" statutes raise questions as to their effectiveness, particularly in terms of the level of compliance. Penalties under such statutes vary, but perhaps the greatest concern with failure to comply with them is the media and public reaction to situations that come to light where there is noncompliance, followed by serious harm to one or more patients. There are no simple answers to questions about the effectiveness of such legislation.

Given the increasing volume and variety of regulation in the health care field, particularly by the states, it is essential that the impact of such reporting legislation be evaluated carefully. Studies of reporting laws, such as those involving venereal disease and suspected child abuse, suggest that compliance is far from universal because of several factors, notably concern about the privacy of the individuals in the case of venereal disease and concern about time-consuming involvement in legal processes related to child abuse.

However, where there is a clear responsibility to report because of the knowledge of the person or institution subject to the requirement, reporting should not be ignored. The implication in the case study that the report will not be made is unfortunate and should not be taken as guidance for the proper way to respond to the legal responsibility.

5.

It would appear that the hospital representatives in the case study were unduly concerned about difficulty of obtaining information about Dr. Morgan's hospitalization, and other evidence relevant to his condition. The burden in a modern set of medical staff bylaws is upon the physician to demonstrate that the doctor continues to meet all the qualifications for medical staff privileges. Therefore, the hospital can request that the physician supply, or give consent to the furnishing of, all appropriate hospital and medical records as a condition of further consideration of the staff appointment.

Thus, the hospital should have demanded that Dr. Morgan authorize East Side General Hospital to furnish a copy of his medical chart to Hope Memorial and that any of Dr. Cooper's records of previous treatment also be provided. In the absence of compliance by Dr. Morgan, the hospital could have taken the position that he had failed to establish, given the circumstances of his hospitalization, that he continued to meet the bylaws' requirements and, therefore, there were grounds to continue the limitation on his opportunity to provide services to his patients in the hospital.

By taking such a stance, the hospital relieves the physician attending the practitioner in question from concerns about maintaining confidentiality in the physician-patient relationship.

6.

The exchange between White and Connors, the administrators of Hope Memorial and East Side General, respectively, as to the content of Dr. Morgan's medical record illustrates the carefulness that frequently is manifested in handling sensitive information involving physicians. The desire to pass on relevant information conflicts with the wish to avoid going on the record officially when the information is derogatory or negative.

Perhaps, if the persons from whom such material was sought were more forthcoming with regard to information that is true and pertinent to decision making, the need for reporting laws of the type involved in the case study would be reduced.

Case 9

Caution—Tactician at Work

PERSONAE

Dr. Barry Bliss, member of the Mary Hamilton Hospital medical staff Executive Committee.
Clarence Coulter, administrator of the Mary Hamilton, protagonist
Fred Gale, an assistant administrator at the Mary Hamilton
Dr. Dennis Lacey, new staff member at the Stonybrook Hospital, protagonist
Dr. Ralph Lawson, medical staff internist, the Mary Hamilton
Frank Morton, deceased former administrator at the Mary Hamilton
Sidney Simon, Coulter's mentor in earlier years
Harry Turner, attorney for the Mary Hamilton
Thomas Williams, administrator of the Stonybrook

Clarence Coulter was swinging his tennis racket in his office while standing and talking on the telephone. Coulter, administrator of the Mary Hamilton Hospital in Morrisville, was an avid tennis player and frequently took his calls while practicing his swing. His office staff and, for that matter, most of the facility's employees, were familiar both with his interest in tennis and his proclivity for practicing his grip and swing while in the hospital. Once, and only once, he had taken his tennis racket to a hospital board meeting. The chairman had told him the hospital did not need an administrator who could not put his recreational pursuits in perspective. Coulter never carried his racket to a board meeting again; in fact, he never even touched it when the chairman was present—or even expected.

He was talking with a physician on the medical staff who, in the past, had been a good source of information about what was stirring in the hospital, particularly among fellow staff members. The physician, Dr. Ralph Lawson, was a well-respected practitioner of internal medicine and a person who never let any conversation pass his ears without paying some attention to it and filing away tidbits for future use. The relationship between Dr. Lawson and Coulter yielded unspoken benefits to both. Coulter received information that otherwise might not reach him until later, if at all, and Dr. Lawson had Coulter looking out for his interests when "perks" or boondoggles came along, such as attendance at a seminar in snow country during the ski season and the administrator was participating in selecting medical staff members to attend at hospital expense.

Dr. Lawson was saying, "I understand that a cardiologist named Dennis Lacey has opened an office midway between Morrisville and Stonybrook and already has been given appointment to the staff at Stonybrook Hospital. He has mentioned to several of the docs on the staff here that he also would be interested in a staff appointment at the Mary Hamilton. From what I hear, there is some concern about Dr. Lacey. It is not clear exactly what brought him, at the age of 40, to relocate in this area if he is as good a doc as he claims he is. Apparently, he told people that he had practiced in Denver but decided to come back East because he had enough living in the West, and that he had some relatives in this area he wanted to be able to see more frequently. Have you gotten an application from him, or has he been in touch with you at all?"

Coulter did not recall any letter or telephone conversation with anyone named Lacey and so told Dr. Lawson. He asked, "Is there anything specific that anyone knows about him, apart from the fact that he is new to the area and has an appointment at Stonybrook already?"

"I don't have any information other than what I have just told you, but I thought I'd let you know that this guy is on the scene and, as far as I'm concerned, my role is over. I want to remind you that your late and unlamented predecessor, Frank Morton, may he rest in peace, once found himself in a lot of difficulty because someone came to town who seemed like a good doctor, was not checked out carefully, and turned out to be a real dog. While I know the medical staff has a lot of responsibility in making recommendations, you and I know that the administrator is going to get blamed if someone like that gets on the staff and creates problems."

"Listen, I appreciate your letting me know and I'll keep my ears open, just as I expect you to, but I'm not going to get into a panic just because a new doctor is in the area, is making some noises about possibly seeking privileges here, and there is some reason to question his background."

"All right, keep swinging that racket, but don't forget that I called if you hear anything from Dr. Lacey."

"I certainly won't forget about it and I appreciate your keeping in touch with me."

* * * * *

The following Saturday Coulter was playing in a tennis tournament at the Racquet Club in Stonybrook that had begun Friday evening. He had entered both the singles and the doubles in the A level. He had done worse than he had expected in the singles, losing his second match, but he and his partner were in the quarterfinals of the doubles with a good chance that they would at least reach the semis, which were to be held Sunday. He was nervously pacing, trying to concentrate on the upcoming match, and sipping from a can of Coke when a slender man, dressed in street clothes, approached him. The man did not look familiar and Coulter, trying to avoid any distractions, glanced away from him. However, the man stepped up next to him and said, "I understand that you're Coulter, the administrator of the Mary Hamilton Hospital in Morrisville."

Coulter was a little taken aback by the remark because he was not thinking at all about his work as he prepared mentally for the match. He said, "Yes, I'm the guy you're talking about. Have you come to see me play and watch my scintillating game?" He said that with a grin, expecting a smile and, perhaps, a quip in return.

The man did not appear to take the remark lightly. He said, "I'm a physician, and I've been wondering whether it would be advisable for me to get an appointment in your hospital. I'm already on the staff at Stonybrook but I expect my practice will bring me into contact with patients who would prefer to go to your institution. Therefore, I was thinking that it might be advisable for me to get privileges at your shop and I wonder if you have a minute, before you get on the court, to chat about my situation."

Coulter was of no mind to continue this conversation. He said, and he was not choosing his words very diplomatically, "I'm sorry. On Saturday and Sunday, unless a problem has come up at the hospital that I'm responsible for, or unless I am attending a meeting in connection with my job, I forget about my work. I'm here in Stonybrook to play tennis and, while I don't want to sound impolite, I am not interested in talking with you or anybody else about a medical staff appointment at the Mary Hamilton right now. As far as I'm concerned, you can call me any day of the work week and I'll be happy to talk with you if I'm in. If you send a letter, I'll respond to it, but please. . . this is not the place to talk business."

The man said, "I guess I have chosen a bad time to talk, please excuse me." He walked off rapidly and Coulter went back to putting himself in the proper frame of mind for doubles.

The tennis was a success. Coulter and his partner won the A level doubles championship cup. That made him feel a lot less upset about his early loss in the singles. In fact, it made him feel so good that he completely forgot about the conversation that had distressed him somewhat Saturday afternoon.

* * * * *

Three weeks later Coulter was buzzed by his receptionist, who told him that a Dr. Lacey was on the phone. Coulter stood up, grabbed his Head, and, with the receiver in the left hand and the racket in the right, moved around the desk while saying, "This is Coulter here."

The voice at the other end sounded vaguely familiar. "When I last talked with you, you told me to reach you at your office and this is, quite frankly, the first chance I've had to call because I have been very busy. My name is Dennis Lacey. I met you at the Racquet Club in Stonybrook and I'd like to talk to you about getting an appointment at Mary Hamilton Hospital."

The administrator realized that he was going to be propositioned—that was the word he liked to use when a physician made inquiries about a medical staff appointment—by a man toward whom he had already an antipathy because he had broken Coulter's concentration before a tennis match.

"Well, I guess we could talk on the phone but I think the best thing would be if you came in to see me and we decided to take a look at the situation sitting around a table, informally. I'm sure sitting down face to face will let us feel more comfortable than talking on the phone."

Coulter was bending his knees and stroking his forehand as he spoke. He had suggested a meeting, having been greatly impressed by a lecture he had attended years before. The lecturer, a trial attorney, had stressed how much could be learned by close visual observation of a prospective witness and Coulter wanted to watch Dr. Lacey closely to see whether he could pick up some useful information.

"I have no objection to that," Dr. Lacey said. "In fact, I welcome your invitation. I would like to come in to talk with you because I have never been inside Mary Hamilton Hospital and that might give me an opportunity to see exactly what you've got. How about next Wednesday?"

Coulter put down the telephone receiver but kept his grip on the racket as he turned the pages in his appointment book. He noted that he was free most of the afternoon the next Wednesday. He had planned to get away for a little tennis late in the day, so he said, "Can you come in sometime around 2:00 because I've got an appointment later in the afternoon."

"Fine with me for 2:30 in the afternoon," Dr. Lacey responded. "I promise that I won't take more than half an hour of your time. Is there anything I should bring with me or send in advance of our meeting?"

"I think it might be good if you sent me a biographical data sheet or curriculum vitae so I'll know something about you. By the way, I understand that you moved here from the West. Do you have any letters that you might have brought with you from the people who worked with you out there?''

''I don't have any letters like that on hand, but there are a few letters that were sent to Stonybrook, and I can get copies of those if you'd like to see them,'' Dr. Lacey replied.

Coulter said, ''Why don't you bring them along. I think it would be good to have them when we meet.''

As soon as the conversation had ended, Coulter buzzed his receptionist and asked her to locate any one of three members of the medical staff Executive Committee he named. The one reached was Dr. Barry Bliss. Coulter said:

''Barry, I want a little help from you. I've made an appointment next Wednesday with some doc named Lacey, who is making noises about getting an appointment here at the hospital. I have agreed to see him but I think it would be good if you are available to join me, either at the start of the meeting, or a few minutes later after I have been able to get a little reading on the situation.

''Just between us, I was warned that this bird was going to make some move toward us and he pissed me off a bit a few weeks ago when he started a conversation with me at the Racquet Club at Stonybrook while I was in the midst of getting revved up for a match. I'm not going to hold that against him, although he certainly showed a lack of taste in bothering me on a Saturday. In any event, can you make it?''

Dr. Bliss answered, ''I can come to your office almost any time in the afternoon that day because I'll be in the hospital anyway. You didn't tell me when you are meeting with this fellow. What time did you have in mind?''

Coulter told him that after Dr. Lacey arrived, he would have his secretary call him to join them. He urged Dr. Bliss to keep his ears open for any remarks staff members might make about Dr. Lacey, and to note who made them.

* * * * *

Of the administrators with whom Coulter had worked during his career, the one who had impressed him the most was Sidney Simon, who had employed him as a second-level assistant shortly after he had received his master's degree. Simon was chief executive of one of the large metropolitan area Jewish hospitals and was highly regarded nationally. Simon frequently had reminded his subordinates when discussing various issues that an administrator must choose a position and find a way to deal with the situation to obtain the result he desired. From Simon's perspective, the administrator knew better than the medical staff and the board what the end result should be in almost every instance, and it was his duty to the institution to find the technique or plan of action by which the proper result could be achieved.

Applying the Simon approach to the appointment of Dr. Lacey to the medical staff meant to Coulter that he would make a decision and, once that was done, he would maneuver in such a fashion that it would become that of the institution. The trick in these matters, he realized, based on what he had learned from Simon, was to function on two levels: (1) as just the hired hand of the board so he would not appear to be usurping the prerogatives of others, and (2) where he would greatly influence all that was done by others without their recognizing what he was doing. He had done this time and again with success at the Mary Hamilton and he had little doubt he could orchestrate almost any situation.

* * * * *

Dr. Lacey's biographical data sheet and copies of two letters sent to Stonybrook Hospital arrived on the Monday before the scheduled meeting. After Coulter looked them over he realized they contained nothing that indicated there would be any particular problems with Dr. Lacey as a physician. However, he had an instinctive feeling that the letters left things unsaid that might not be favorable to the physician. Both letters merely stated that Dr. Lacey had been on the medical staffs of the two hospitals in the West and that he had never had his privileges to practice suspended or revoked during his service there. There were no statements attesting to any specific competencies or contributions to the hospitals, or any other specific matters. The administrator drew the conclusion that it would be better for him and the hospital if Dr. Lacey were not appointed to the staff until he had practiced in the area for at least a year or two. By then the hospital would have had an opportunity to assess his performance in practice, particularly with regard to his medical activities at Stonybrook. Coulter toyed with the idea of calling one of the hospitals in the Denver area but decided that this was premature. At the least, he felt he should wait until he had his meeting with Dr. Lacey.

Dr. Lacey arrived promptly on Wednesday and after a few minutes they were joined by Dr. Bliss, whom Coulter had briefed. The plan was for the two to say as little as possible and to find a way to get Dr. Lacey to do most of the talking.

Dr. Lacey put his cards on the table rather rapidly, saying he wanted an appointment on the staff and desired to have cardiology privileges, although he realized that since he had only one year of cardiology specialty training in addition to two years of internal medicine residency there were certain cardiology procedures he was not prepared to undertake. He talked at some length about the range of cardiology practice he had developed in the West and said that his privileges at Stonybrook accommodated his desires for cardiology.

Coulter asked only a few questions. One concerned whether Dr. Lacey had been in a partnership or other group arrangement with other physicians while he was in the West, a second involved whether he planned to join or affiliate with any local group, and a third was why he had chosen to leave the Denver area and return to the East.

Dr. Lacey responded to the effect that he had practiced in a partnership for a while, that he had no plans at the current time to join a group but that he had made some coverage arrangements for his patients that were working out well with a group, and that there was a possibility he might join it eventually. As the reason for leaving the West, he said he was originally from upstate New York, had relatives throughout a good deal of the East, and wanted to keep in closer touch with his family than was possible when he was in Denver.

Dr. Bliss didn't ask any questions although he did make a few comments in response to Dr. Lacey's statements. As the conversation was winding down Coulter said, "You told me that you wanted to see our operation and I have arranged with one of our assistant administrators to give you a grand tour if you have the time. Would you like him to take you around now?"

"That would be fine. I think that I've told you all I can and I would like to see the hospital while I'm here. I would like to thank both of you for the time you have spent with me and I'll be in touch some time soon."

Lacey shook hands with Coulter and Bliss. Fred Gale, an assistant administrator, came in and led Dr. Lacey out on the tour of the hospital. After they had left, Coulter asked, "What do you think, Barry?"

Dr. Bliss paused, then answered, "I see no reason from what we heard for us to reject him for an appointment. Of course, we really didn't learn much about his practice. We don't know why he left the group he said he was part of in Denver, and I have an uneasy feeling about him."

Coulter mentally agreed with that assessment but he did not say anything to indicate he had any reservations. Rather, he said, "If he applies we will treat him as we would any other applicant for medical staff appointment." As he said those words there was a very fleeting smile on his face. Dr. Bliss noted the smile and, while he said nothing, gave it substantial meaning.

Dr. Lacey returned to Coulter's office an hour later and thanked him for making Gale available. He said he was impressed with the physical plant and what appeared to be a very efficient operation but he did not ask for a staff appointment application form.

* * * * *

Absorbed in many matters of concern to the hospital, Coulter promptly forgot about his meeting with Dr. Lacey. The hospital was giving preliminary thoughts to a corporate restructuring, a union was making noises about collective bargaining for the nonprofessional employees, and the administrator was engaged in tedious negotiations for the purchase of a nearby piece of county-owned land that he believed the institution should acquire to protect itself from encroachment by a use inconsistent with his long-range ideas about its future.

Three weeks later Coulter was scheduled to play tennis late in the afternoon with Harry Turner, the hospital's attorney, to be followed by dinner, at which there would be general discussion of "big picture" matters concerning the hospital. They had long adhered to an unspoken rule that they would not talk hospital business until after they had played. Turner, who was several years younger, usually beat the administrator but only after a fierce struggle. Coulter greatly enjoyed the competition because it helped sharpen his game.

As Coulter joined Turner at courtside—the pair on their court wanted to finish a final game—Coulter thrust a piece of paper into Turner's hands and said, "Take a look at this. Those dummies have done it once again. What do you think Harry?"

Turner glanced briefly at the letter and saw that it concerned the hospital.

"Now wait a minute," he said, "I thought we are here to play tennis. We can talk about hospital matters later."

"I know we can, but I am just so mad I have to show you this now." Turner read the letter rapidly. The key sentence in the letter, which was addressed to Dr. Lacey, stated:

> The Department of Medicine has considered your qualifications and has voted unanimously that you could not be granted cardiology privileges at the hospital, based on your limited cardiology training.

Turner asked, "Has this fellow Lacey applied for a medical staff appointment?"

"That's why they are such dummies. Dr. Lacey came to me for a meeting and I discussed with him—Barry Bliss, who I thought had more sense than this letter indicates, was present—and the end result was that it was up to Dr. Lacey to make an application, although we didn't talk specifically about it. The only reason I knew about the letter is that my good friend Ralph Lawson told me it already had gone out and I was able to get a copy just before leaving the hospital."

Turner said nothing, and the pair went on the court to play. Turner whipped Coulter badly, with the latter winning only eight games in three sets. At dinner later the administrator blamed the letter for a loss of concentration that hampered his play. Turner sympathized with him but could not resist the opportunity to give him the needle.

"I thought they taught you when you were studying management that a good manager focuses on the matter at hand. Once we got on the court the matter at hand was tennis, not some physician's staff appointment. Don't you think Jimmy Connors has other things to think about besides tennis sometimes?"

Coulter was not amused.

Most of the discussion during the meal was devoted to the matters Coulter had planned to bring up, but several times they returned to the Lacey letter. Turner pointed out that the Department of Medicine's action could create difficulty in the event Dr. Lacey were denied an appointment later because it would appear to indicate that the decision had been made before a review of the information in his application and of other data from the sources usually contacted in conformity with medical staff bylaws procedures. In counseling Coulter, Turner said,

"Let me make two proposals to you, both of which I think you ought to consider seriously. First, I urge that you send a letter to Dr. Lacey tomorrow that blandly says that you noted that he had failed to request, and therefore was not given, a medical staff application form, and that you are sending one along with the letter. Make it clear in your letter that his application will be reviewed as would be any other one received by the hospital for medical staff appointment. Don't mention the letter from the Department of Medicine at all.

"The second suggestion is that, from now on, you arrange for one of your administrative staff to attend all meetings of the medical staff departments. I am certain that some of the doctors will be upset when one of your aides is present but I think the lesson brought home by this letter business is that the medical staff does not have quite the grasp of some issues that it should, particularly because of the legal considerations that may enter into some of the actions it recommends or takes."

Coulter agreed to follow both recommendations and to send Turner a copy of his letter to Dr. Lacey.

* * * * *

Coulter decided on his strategy for dealing with Dr. Lacey with respect to the staff appointment. It was the practice at Mary Hamilton Hospital for the administration to hold staff appointment application forms until they were complete before turning them over to the Credentials Committee. Coulter decided he did not want the issue of Dr. Lacey's staff appointment to get into the recommendation and decision process until the physician had practiced for a considerably longer time in the area so that some conclusions could be reached as to his current competency, ethical standards, etc.

What Coulter proposed to do if Dr. Lacey did apply was to take as much time as he could as part of the process of determining when the application was complete. He planned to send letters not only to persons given as references on the application form but also to others whose names he would obtain from Dr. Lacey as well as from other contacts he might develop, and that this information-gathering process would consume three to six months. He felt fairly secure that, in spite of the fact that the medical staff bylaws provided for relatively short periods for Credentials Committee and medical staff Executive

Committee consideration and recommendation, by holding off on presenting the application under the guise that it was not complete enough for the panel to review, he could avoid technical violations of the bylaws and still achieve his objective.

Several days after the administrator sent his letter to Dr. Lacey he called Dr. Bliss in for an informal discussion of the situation. Dr. Bliss contended that he should bear no blame for the Department of Medicine's letter because he was not the chairman and that since several members had indicated serious reservations about Dr. Lacey's minimal training in cardiology, the content was fundamentally correct. Although Coulter pointed out several times that formal communications with a physician indicating a negative view respecting an appointment, before the doctor had even submitted an application, might prejudice the hospital's position at some later date if an appointment eventually were to be denied and litigation were to ensue, Dr. Bliss apparently felt that little harm had been done.

"I think the letter gave Dr. Lacey a signal," he said. "I was not the source of the C.V. that the department had when it discussed Lacey. Frankly, I don't know how the department obtained a copy of it, but the most important element to me was that on its face, it indicated very little preparation for cardiology privileges."

"Listen, I talked with our attorney the day I learned about the letter," Coulter responded. "I was really annoyed. From what he told me, all of you may have laid yourselves open to some kind of legal problems on a conspiracy or restraint-of-trade theory. When I sent an application form to Dr. Lacey the day after I learned of the letter, I was trying to pull your chestnuts out of the fire."

"I don't want the Department of Medicine or any other group in the hospital sending out any letters dealing with appointments unless they have been cleared with me, and I probably will have those kinds of letters cleared with our attorney if I have any questions about their content. From now on, one of my people is going to attend every department meeting. . . at least until I am convinced no foul-ups will occur."

When he finished, Dr. Bliss appeared considerably chastened. Seeking to soften his comments, the administrator added, "Look, a mistake was made. I have tried to prevent harm from that mistake. I am not trying to put blame on anyone now. What's done is done. The hospital and the medical staff just have to make sure that we don't prejudice our situation by getting sued for no good reason. We've all learned a lesson, and I hope the lesson is not forgotten."

* * * * *

More than a month passed before Dr. Lacey submitted his application form to Mary Hamilton Hospital. Coulter reviewed it very carefully. He noted that the physician had listed three hospitals as institutions where he had practiced and that he had been in residency programs at two medical centers. The administrator let another three weeks go by, then wrote to Dr. Lacey asking him to indicate persons Coulter should contact at the hospitals and the medical centers where he had trained. Dr. Lacey wrote back within a week giving two names at each hospital and the names of the individuals who had directed the residency programs. Coulter waited two more weeks, then wrote to the named persons, asking them to complete a form developed at the hospital for comments on applicants for staff appointment. Two of the forms were returned within two weeks but none of the other persons responded.

The administrator waited a month after his initial mailing, then sent follow-ups to those who had not answered. When Dr. Lacey called during that period, Coulter told him that the gathering of information was going slowly because some of the individuals the physician had mentioned had not responded. He assured Dr. Lacey that, if necessary, he would attempt to telephone the individuals to stress the need for their comments. The follow-up mailing only elicited one more response, and after waiting two weeks from the date he received the last reply, he called those from whom nothing had been received in writing.

He learned that Dr. Lacey's medical residency program director was now at another academic medical center. Two physicians and one hospital administrator no longer were at the institutions to which the letters had been mailed and all he could obtain were leads as to where they might be reached. He received little information in the telephone conversations from those he did contact; they told him they preferred not to complete the forms but declined to give any specific reasons.

Two weeks after the telephone calls, Coulter mailed comment forms to the individuals who now were at other locations and who apparently had never received the originals. He then telephoned Dr. Lacey and told him the investigation was continuing and that he needed additional names because several of the persons listed initially were unwilling to comment in writing. He also asked for the names of two of the physicians who had been in the group with which Dr. Lacey had practiced in the West. The physician supplied additional names and such addresses as he could provide. Coulter recognized that Dr. Lacey was unhappy with the slow progress and wondered what he might do.

Coulter didn't have to wonder long. Three days later he received a letter from Dr. Lacey requesting that he be granted temporary privileges while his appointment was being reviewed. He specifically requested some noninvasive cardiology privileges and wrote that he frequently had performed those procedures in the West and currently was doing most of them at Stonybrook Hospital.

The administrator had anticipated a request for temporary privileges and had developed a plan of action or, perhaps better, inaction. According to the medical staff bylaws, the decision on granting temporary privileges in these circumstances depended upon joint action of the administrator, the president of the medical staff, and the department chairman under whose general supervision the physician would practice.

Coulter decided he would not even contact the two physicians but handle the matter himself. He had two reasons: (1) he didn't want to stir up members of the medical staff about Dr. Lacey's application and (2) he wanted to forestall what he regarded as any silly action by members of the Department of Medicine. He rationalized his decision on the basis that, because any one of the three could veto temporary privileges and he as one of the three was not ready to grant them at this time—in effect, he was vetoing the application for the time being—there was no need to consult the others.

He responded in a long letter that said relatively little. Its key point was that, although temporary privileges could be granted while an application was pending, given that Dr. Lacey already was practicing in another hospital in the area, there was no particular need for providing temporary privileges at this time. Coulter assured the physician that, if there were particular patients who needed services that could be provided only at Mary Hamilton Hospital and were not available at Stonybrook, Dr. Lacey could request temporary privileges for such patients on an individual basis and the hospital would be willing to respond speedily.

* * * * *

Sixth months had now passed since Dr. Lacey's application form had reached his desk. Coulter was proud of the way he had maneuvered to postpone consideration of it by any medical staff committee. He decided he would do nothing further officially until he received another letter or telephone call from Dr. Lacey. At that point he would propose that, in the interest of speeding the application process—Coulter wanted to give the illusion that he was attempting to help Dr. Lacey—Mary Hamilton Hospital now was going to solicit information concerning his practice at Stonybrook. This, Coulter would indicate, would provide his institution with current information on the nature and quality of Dr. Lacey's present performance and that, if necessary, review of specific charts could be undertaken rapidly. By taking this tack, Coulter hoped that if there were some problems or questions on Dr. Lacey's performance at Stonybrook, the physician might decide that discretion was the better part of valor and withdraw his application. Even though the administrator was not planning to take any official action, he thought that it would be useful to get some kind of informal appraisal from Stonybrook as soon as he could.

Coulter telephoned Thomas Williams, the Stonybrook administrator. After an exchange of greetings, Coulter started talking generally about the need for hospital administrators to exchange information informally to protect the interests of their respective institutions concerning physicians who sought or held medical staff appointments. Williams could not tell whether Coulter was about to seek information or whether he had some useful piece of information about a physician on the Stonybrook staff. He mumbled "Yes" and "That's right" several times while Coulter's monologue on responsibilities and duties continued.

Having, in a sense, set Williams up to be frank and candid, Coulter then said, "I understand that a Dr. Lacey who has applied for privileges at the Mary Hamilton has been a member of the staff at your shop for at least a year. We are in the process of evaluating his application and I think it probably would be very useful to us to find out how he looks to you and the folks at your place. Everything you tell me will be kept in the strictest confidence. I won't make any notes about our discussion and no one here knows that I'm even making this call."

Williams was a bit disappointed. He had begun to anticipate that he was going to pick up information about someone on his staff and now he realized he was becoming a source, rather than a recipient, of what could be sensitive material. He said, "I hope that the next time the situation is reversed and I need something from you. . . that you will give it to me straight from the shoulder."

"Wait a minute Tom," Coulter interjected. "Have I ever not given you information about a doctor or anyone when you asked for it? Did I ever hold out on you?"

"Well, Clarence, I think it is fair to say that you have never withheld anything from me when I've asked. However, I can't recall that I ever talked to you about a physician. The only people I ever asked you about were nurses or technical people who had left your place, or were considering doing so, and were applying for jobs here. I think you realize that is a little different from a question about the medical staff."

"I suppose that's so. But I haven't ever failed to give you information that was honest. You'll have to admit that."

"I don't want to beat this into the ground," Williams said. "I've talked to a number of administrators at times about applicants to our medical staff and it has been like pulling teeth. I'm not the kind of guy who holds back information and the reason I brought it up is that I want to be confident that you're not that kind of guy, either."

"I'm not. I know how you feel about those guys who hardly say anything and still act like they are parting with the crown jewels. You can count on me to give you the straight scoop when you need it."

Williams then began to talk about Dr. Lacey. "I haven't heard any complaints about him from anybody. Not from nurses, not from technicians, and not from any of the docs here. Apparently he keeps his nose clean, doesn't get anybody excited, and minds his own business. Frankly, I don't know what he does professionally. I can tell you that if he was screwing up I would have heard of it by now."

"Tom, can you check a little more deeply for me? I would like to know particularly what he is doing in cardiology. He has told us that he has fairly extensive privileges in cardiology and I think that some of our guys don't believe he is qualified for much, if anything, in cardiology based on his limited training. Of course, he may have done a lot before he came to Stonybrook but I'd like to know what he is doing in your place."

"I'll take a look-see and get back to you when I can. By the way, has anybody given you any information that makes you suspicious about our friend Lacey? A few of your guys practice here also and if they know something that I should know and they've told you but haven't told me, I'd sure like to know it now."

"Don't worry, if I had anything I'd be happy to give it to you."

Coulter had thought of mentioning the letter sent by his Department of Medicine months before but decided that this was not the time. He was afraid Williams would consider he had failed to control the department. While Coulter didn't feel that he was at all responsible for the letter, he feared that Williams might see it a little differently and that might make him more reticent about sharing information.

* * * * *

A week went by before Williams called Coulter. "I have a few items to mention about Dr. Lacey. It appears that although he has a fair amount of noninvasive cardiology privileges, he has used them very little. In fact, in the last six months or so he hasn't done anything that we don't generally allow our straight medical people to do. He used his privileges a fair amount when he first started here. I didn't turn up anything that tells me he was inadequate. But, in any event, he's just practicing internal medicine here now and he uses cardiology consultants to about the same extent as anyone else with internal medicine privileges without any specialty stuff in cardiology.

"Actually, he appears to be very cautious. I have one interesting clue about what may be happening. He has gotten pretty close with the members of one of our better groups. Those guys cover for him when he is out of town or taking time off from his practice. One of the people in that group is a boarded cardiologist and Lacey gives him almost all of his consults. It may be that he is sucking up to them a little and hopes he'll be able to join the group, although I haven't heard anything along that line from anybody. I think it is a shrewd move on Dr. Lacey's part to send the business over, particularly if he thinks he might be able to fit in with that group one of these days. They have a good rep professionally and they never give me any trouble."

Coulter was very pleased by the information and expressed his gratitude. He then reviewed the situation mentally. He decided he was in a position to turn

Dr. Lacey away without having the physician kick up a serious fuss. Up to this point he had shared his delaying tactics scenario with no one. Now he felt it would be advisable to mention it at least to Turner, the hospital's attorney.

* * * * *

He invited Turner to join him for dinner after tennis. Coulter was in excellent spirits at dinner that day because he had achieved one of his infrequent victories over Turner and the attorney hadn't advanced any physical complaint or business pressure as an excuse for his loss. The administrator summarized the maneuvers he had made to keep Dr. Lacey on hold for half a year and in so doing had exhibited pride in his accomplishment. Coulter expected approbation.

Turner told Coulter that nothing he had done seemed to have put the hospital in any serious danger if Dr. Lacey became so fed up that he consulted an attorney, with the expectation that he could get help in court. But the attorney expressed some reservations. He sought to get across the point that, while the delaying tactic had worked, there was some question in his mind as to whether Coulter was usurping responsibilities placed in others by the hospital's corporate and medical staff documents. As he talked in this vein, Coulter played with his teaspoon and, although he did not interrupt, he became more and more agitated.

After Turner finished Coulter said, "You are not the manager of the Mary Hamilton and responsible for all that takes place there. I am. The more problems that I let get into the hands of others, the greater difficulty I have in influencing what takes place. I can't fight on three or four fronts at once. I know there was no way the medical staff would recommend favorably on Dr. Lacey's application for cardiology privileges. Under the bylaws, if there was an adverse recommendation on cardiology, he would have requested a hearing, and you and I know from the experience of other hospitals, as well as ours, that this is an upsetting experience and it could cost us a lot of time, effort, and bucks.

"Last year, when I was at the meeting of the American Hospital Association, I spoke with an administrator from California. He had just had a hearing involving a physician that ran for a total of at least 30 hours. To play it safe—to try to avoid a court's getting involved later—they hired some lawyer to serve as the hearing officer and the son-of-a-bitch charged them $200 an hour for presiding and another $1,500 for writing up the decision of the hearing committee. According to the administrator the decision was only two pages long, but this lawyer told him, when he sent the bill, that he had to spend time meeting with the members of the committee to find out exactly what they had decided and their reasons for doing so. All we have spent out of pocket so far on Dr. Lacey is a couple of bucks for telephone calls and postage."

Turner had reddened a bit during Coulter's remarks. He then asked, "What is the next step in your grand design?"

"It's very simple. One of these days Dr. Lacey is going to call me and I am going to invite him to come over and have coffee with me and I'm going to lay it on the line with him."

"Pray tell, what does that mean?"

"Very simply," Coulter said, "I'm going to tell him that he hasn't a chance of getting cardiology privileges. I am going to tell him that he hasn't been practicing cardiology at Stonybrook and, therefore, we have no basis for evaluating him favorably with regard to the privileges he seeks. Thus, the best I can see him getting is an appointment for internal medicine only, and I am prepared to put it in such a way that getting those privileges may be a struggle that he probably would be better off avoiding.

"I plan to let him know that we know he is hoping to get involved with a group that practices only at Stonybrook and that he will have some difficulties in getting coverage for any of his patients he admits to the Mary Hamilton. I will also hint to him that, if members of the group he is playing around with at Stonybrook were to apply for privileges here, it will take a lot of time to check them out and that it probably wouldn't be worth the effort."

"Do you think that will get rid of Dr. Lacey?"

"You betcha it will. I know these doctors well enough, and if Dr. Lacey has a fuss here he won't look that good to the physicians he is romancing up at Stonybrook. Also, those doctors at Stonybrook are unlikely to even make a move to get on the staff here in order to help Dr. Lacey. Remember, I am going to be very polite, interested, helpful, sympathetic, and all that stuff, when I talk with him. If I do it right, he is going to consider me almost a friend. I'll be talking to him almost like an uncle."

"I'm glad you told me all this, although I really don't see why it was even necessary."

"Harry, you are our attorney and I like to keep you informed. If you were to tell me that we're in a difficult position legally, I'd be looking to you for advice. I thought I would check with you to find out whether we were in a difficult position. From what you have said the hospital is in pretty good shape regarding Dr. Lacey. That makes me happy. I haven't looked to you for management advice. That's my ball game. Some of the administrators I know check with their lawyer every time they go to the bathroom. I consider that poor upbringing. I don't hide things from you. I just don't ask you to tell me what to do when I can make up my mind for myself."

During the rest of the dinner they talked of other things and did not return to Dr. Lacey.

* * * * *

Several days later, Dr. Lacey made the telephone call that Coulter had been expecting. The administrator invited Dr. Lacey to visit with him, saying he had some news that would interest the physician. When Dr. Lacey arrived, Coulter was very polite. He said at the outset that he wanted to level with him as a physician. He began a long monologue explaining all the difficulties he had encountered in obtaining information. He explained that he had learned of the very limited use of the cardiology privileges at Stonybrook and predicted that the Mary Hamilton medical staff Executive Committee recommendation to the hospital board on cardiology privileges almost certainly would be adverse to Dr. Lacey. Then, as tactfully as he could, he suggested that it would be to Dr. Lacey's advantage to withdraw his application by writing a letter saying that at the current time he was not interested in an appointment at Mary Hamilton Hospital. In his remarks, Coulter virtually drafted the letter he wanted Dr. Lacey to send.

While Coulter was speaking, Dr. Lacey showed some signs of discomfort but did not interrupt once. Finally, after the administrator had finished, Dr. Lacey responded.

"I can read the situation. You don't have to worry about me. You had me jump through a few hoops, and I know that's part of the game. Frankly, I am not looking for a fight with this hospital. I don't know if I could win one or not, but I'm not going to get into one anyway. You're right, I am not doing much cardiology today and the way things look I won't be doing much in the future. I get along well with the people up at Stonybrook and I don't want to go any place where I am not wanted.

"You are a pretty shrewd guy, I grant that. I was told that you were by a few friends as soon as I told people that I was applying for an appointment here. I just want you to know that I'm not a lousy doctor. I came back from the West not because of problems but because I wanted to be in this area for legitimate reasons. I would bet that you haven't got anything about me that would stand up as a reason not to appoint me to the staff here. There are some doctors who would fight just for the sake of showing they're not going to be pushed around. I don't like to waste my money like that."

Dr. Lacey stood up to leave. He did not extend his hand to shake the one offered by Coulter, who also had risen. "Just one more thing," Dr. Lacey said. "I don't want to hear from anyone that you did any bragging about how you kept me away from the Mary Hamilton. That would get me really mad."

Dr. Lacey walked to the door of Coulter's office, opened it, and left without glancing back.

Coulter reached his phone console and contacted his secretary. "Have Fred Gale get in here as soon as he can, I've got something I want to tell him." Then he picked up his racket and started practicing his backhand swing.

Commentary

1.

Most people dislike the Coulters of this world. At the same time, many of these same individuals grudgingly admire their results. Coulter justified his course of action, at least to himself; he succeeded in preventing Dr. Lacey's application from requiring a medical staff recommendation and action by the hospital board, which probably would have made for a long and troubling series of proceedings. While the case study ends before his conversation with Fred Gale, it can be imagined that he recounted his handling of the Lacey application with pride and satisfaction.

2.

Not infrequently, a physician considering applying for a medical staff appointment seeks informal advice or opinions from the hospital administrator, medical staff leaders, and even board members. Those contacted must avoid strong positive or negative responses.

Discretion is essential in responding to a likely applicant. The letter from the Department of Medicine is an excellent example of what not to do. If there are specific requirements in the bylaws that the physician does not meet, these certainly can be mentioned but anything indicating a decision already has been made, or certainly will be, is uncalled for. Letters and other communications of the sort sent by the Department of Medicine go out far too frequently. Coulter's action to undo the damage by sending his letter and an application form, after talking with the hospital's attorney, cannot be faulted.

3.

Physicians pursue different strategies in requesting clinical privileges as part of the initial appointment process. Some believe they should ask for as great a range of privileges as might possibly be granted, assuming they will get somewhat less than they request. Others tend to keep their initial requests modest to avoid giving any grounds for adverse action, with the expectation that, after a period of competent practice at the hospital, there will be receptivity to gradual expansion of their privileges.

Today, because of the high degree of specialization in medicine, and the trend toward reserving certain areas for physicians who have contracts with the hospital, assignment of privileges is a complex matter. For many physicians, admitting privileges are subordinate in importance to the range of services they can provide to patients they admit and to other patients who are, or might be, referred to them by staff doctors for specific diagnostic and treatment procedures.

In this context, the need to justify restraints on competition through assignments of privileges become more and more of an issue. For example, at many institutions general surgeons are finding their privileges being circumscribed, at least in part in response to pressures from various surgical specialists. In medicine, physicians with subspecialties in respiratory and cardiology areas are seeking to limit the range of privileges granted family practitioners and internists without extensive subspecialty training.

Looking at the foregoing in terms of Dr. Lacey, his prospects for cardiology privileges would be very limited at many hospitals today unless he obtained further training. There is considerable reluctance to seriously consider and evaluate prior experience in some specialty areas if the applicant lacks extensive graduate training when physicians with more extensive training in these areas, and a track record, are members of the hospital medical staff.

Concluding Observations

Governing Board—Medical Staff—Chief Executive Officer: The Eternal Triangle (Tangle)

In the era of simplicity for hospitals that ended less than two decades ago, one of the verities of their organization was the triangle. Ordinarily it was an equilateral triangle, with the governing board at the apex. The other two corners were the medical staff and the administrator respectively (Figure 1).

This simple organizational diagram was used time and time again at institutes and seminars for the hospital field and found its way frequently into articles and other publications.

Using the triangle to explain the nature of hospital organization, and placing the governing board at the apex, meant that the board had the ultimate legal and moral authority and responsibility for the functioning of the institution. The solid lines leading down to the medical staff and the administrator meant that the board was supreme in the organization and that it controlled or directed the others in the performance of their functions. The triangle placed the medical staff and the administrator on the same level, but a lower one, in relation to the governing board.

Whether this actually was the organizational situation at most hospitals in the 1940s, 1950s, and into the 1960s, during the age of simplicity, is not readily apparent. While in a technical sense the governing board might perceive the administrator as being on the same level as the medical staff, there were, and perhaps still are, hospitals where the actual structure, as distinguished from the one represented on paper, could best be shown with the medical staff at the apex of the triangle, the governing board at a lower level, and the administrator at a very acute angle at the bottom of the figure (Figure 2). The triangle would not be equilateral; it would be isosceles, with a very long hypotenuse connecting the medical staff and the administrator.

Figure 1 Hospitals' Old Eternal Triangle

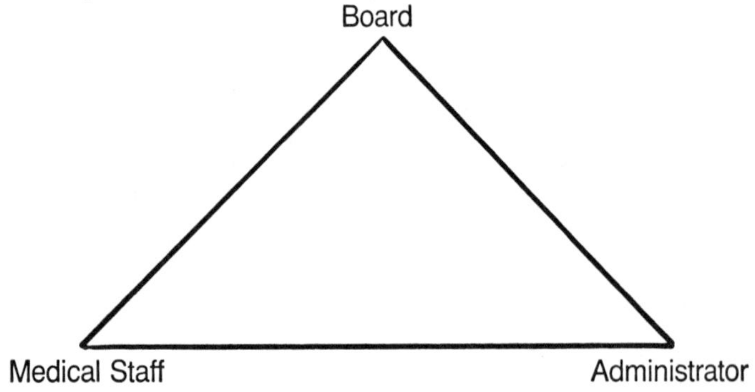

Figure 2 The Old Triangle—Realistically

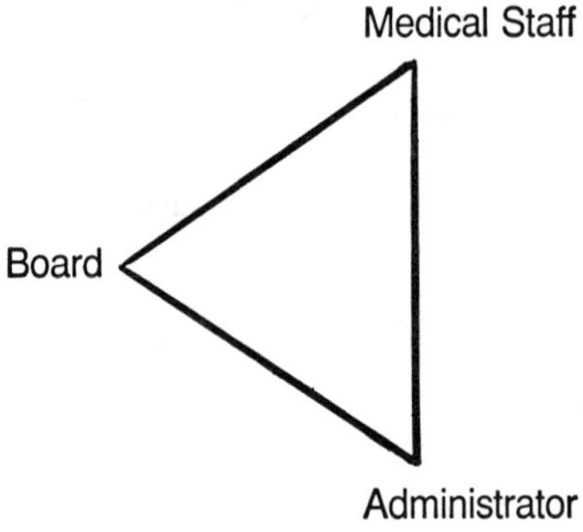

Today a simple triangle to represent hospital relationships just won't do, even if only the formal structure is considered. In most hospitals, the relationships among the governing board, the medical staff, and the administration are too complex. This is particularly true where members of the medical staff serve as voting members of the governing board; where the chief executive officer serves as a member of that board; and where there is a salaried medical director, whose functions substantially affect the performance and activities of the medical staff, who reports nominally at best to the chief executive officer, but who essentially is the agent of the governing board for medical staff oversight and leadership.

In seeking to understand better the relationships among these three elements, it is essential to review the sources or bases for stating that the ultimate authority and responsibility reside in the governing board. There are at least three legal bases for stating the extent of the board's authority and responsibility:

1. There is the explicit or implicit statement in state statutes and/or state agency regulations on the subject. In practically every state where hospitals are licensed or regulated in one form or another by state government, the position of the governing board at the apex of the simplicity triangle is stated.
2. The Medicare Conditions of Participation, the language of which has been borrowed in considerable measure from the Joint Commission on Accreditation of Hospitals principles and standards, recognize the primacy of the governing board and its ultimate authority and responsibility.
3. The developing case law includes numerous instances in which hospitals have been held liable for the harm suffered by patients because of the institutions' failures adequately to review, supervise, and monitor the qualifications and performance of medical staff members. Recognition of hospital responsibility and liability in such circumstances is expanding.

The need for hospitals to respond to these legal developments suggests—realistically, commands—that their governing boards establish and use review and appraisal techniques for applicants to, and members of, medical staffs. These should be embodied in hospital documents, including the institution's bylaws; the medical staff's bylaws, rules, and regulations; and perhaps other documents as well. These documents must clearly set forth the responsibilities and functions of the governing board, medical staff, and administrator.

The case studies and commentaries present both explicitly and implicitly a host of suggestions as to the appropriate content of hospital documents.

The authors and the editor believe that the importance of the role of hospital documents in avoiding or minimizing medical staff problems cannot be overstated. While history and institutional dynamics substantially affect the particulars of the process by which such documents are drafted, refined, and eventually adopted, it is crucial that the process take place. The hospital's attorney can be a facilitator in the process, in addition to being simply the drafter of the documents.

And, with the lack of humility that some believe is characteristic of attorneys, the authors and the editor urge that the contribution of the attorney be sought at the very outset of the process.

About the Editor

NATHAN HERSHEY is Professor of Health Law at the Graduate School of Public Health, University of Pittsburgh, and is counsel to the law firm of Markel, Schafer, & Means, P.A., in Pittsburgh. Professor Hershey received his B.A. degree from New York University in 1950 and his LL.B. from Harvard Law School in 1953. He is a member of the Pennsylvania, District of Columbia (inactive), and New York bars. He has served as a board member and as president (1972) of the American Society of Hospital Attorneys and as a board member and as president (1980) of the Society of Hospital Attorneys of Western Pennsylvania. He was elected a member of the Institute of Medicine, National Academy of Sciences, in 1972. He has served as a member of the State Board of Medical Education and Licensure of Pennsylvania, the Legal Issues Panel of the Secretary's Commission on Medical Malpractice, DHEW, and as a consultant to, or member of, various public and private committees and agencies at the local, state, and national level.

Professor Hershey was one of the original authors of the *Hospital Law Manual and Quarterly Service* and serves as senior adviser to this Aspen Systems Corporation publication. He is a member of the faculty of the Aspen Systems Corporation "Medical Staff Law and Bylaws" and "Consent Practices" seminars. He has authored more than 150 journal articles. In 1969, Professor Hershey, with Stanley H. Bushkoff, M.D., wrote *Informed Consent Study,* and in 1976, with Robert D. Miller, wrote *Human Experimentation and the Law,* both published by Aspen Systems Corporation.